The DASH Diet for Beginners

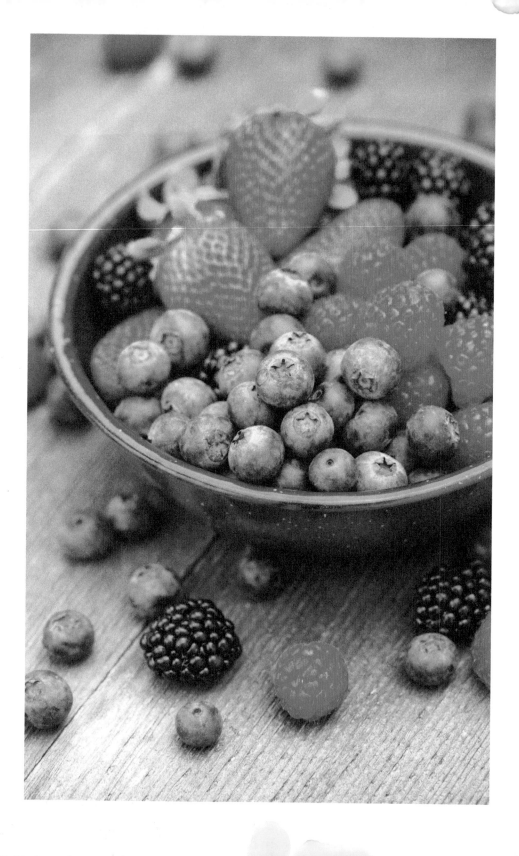

The
DASH Diet
for Beginners

THE GUIDE TO GETTING STARTED

SONOMA PRESS

Contents

Introduction vii

PART **ONE**

Understanding the DASH Diet

Chapter One What Is the DASH Diet? 3

Chapter Two Why the DASH Diet Works 12

PART **TWO**

DASH Diet Health Plan

Chapter Three DASH Diet for High Blood Pressure/Hypertension 19

Chapter Four DASH Diet for Weight Loss 24

Chapter Five DASH Diet for Optimal Health 30

PART **THREE**

Transitioning to the DASH Diet

Chapter Six Tips for Planning Your DASH Diet 35

Chapter Seven DASH Diet Food Groups 43

Chapter Eight Ten Steps for Success 48

PART **FOUR**

DASH Diet in Action

Chapter Nine DASH Diet Eating Guide 55

Chapter Ten DASH-Friendly Cooking Methods 59

Chapter Eleven 30-Day Meal Plan for Health and Weight Loss 62

PART **FIVE**

150 DASH Recipes

Chapter Twelve DASH Breakfasts 87

Chapter Thirteen DASH Lunches 131

Chapter Fourteen DASH Snacks and Appetizers 183

Chapter Fifteen DASH Dinners 225

Chapter Sixteen DASH Desserts 273

Appendix: Shopping and Dining on the DASH Diet 315

Glossary 325

References 328

Index 330

Introduction

Have you been casting around for a sustainable way to lose weight and improve your health—not to mention feel better—that doesn't involve trendy gimmicks, dubious pills, or hunger pangs? If you're like millions of Americans who diet each year, you're ready to trade in faddish schemes and make-believe results for something lasting and real. Enter the DASH diet. With its focus on eating an abundant array of quality, nutrient-rich ingredients, it's ideal for those who have followed other plans and failed to see long-term results. And because you won't be left with that panicky feeling of deprivation—or the sneaking sense that you're rationing your own food—it's easy to make this plan a permanent part of your life. Besides that, the DASH diet goes beyond weight loss to reduce high blood pressure and lower the risk of cancer, diabetes, and osteoporosis—which makes the added benefits just icing on the proverbial cake. (And, yes, desserts are allowed. But more on that later.)

Health concerns related to diet and lifestyle are at an all-time high, and it's no wonder: annual statistics compiled by the American Heart Association reveal that as of 2013, nearly half of all Americans over the age of twenty are overweight or obese. Of the 154.7 million people who fall into these categories, 78.4 million—one in four Americans—are classified as obese, with a body mass index (BMI) of 30 or higher.

Who Is to Blame for these Staggering Statistics?

We can wag our fingers at the standard American diet, with its empty, high-calorie foods rife with unhealthful fat, salt, and sugars. The majority of these same, overly processed foods are also completely devoid of good, heart-healthy fats. To make matters worse, those who consume these foods as a regular part of their diet are not getting enough fiber, nor are they taking in adequate vitamins and minerals.

If you're like most people, you've tried dieting at some point: you've restricted calories, you've eliminated entire food groups, you've even resorted to bizarre potions like lemon juice, cayenne pepper, and maple syrup. Diet plans like these can bring the illusion of success—they often result in immediate weight loss simply because the body is starving; however, once the body snaps out of starvation mode and normal eating resumes, those lost pounds return, often bringing even more weight gain with them.

The DASH diet is different from weight-loss plans that may have let you down in the past. In this book, you'll learn how you can shed pounds and improve your health without having to give up your favorite foods or spend excessive hours exercising. Steps for success, delicious recipes, and tips for adopting healthful habits are included here to ensure that you have all the tools you need to meet your goals—this time, for real.

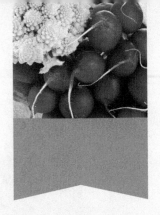

PART ONE

Understanding the DASH Diet

Chapter One What Is the DASH Diet?

Chapter Two Why the DASH Diet Works

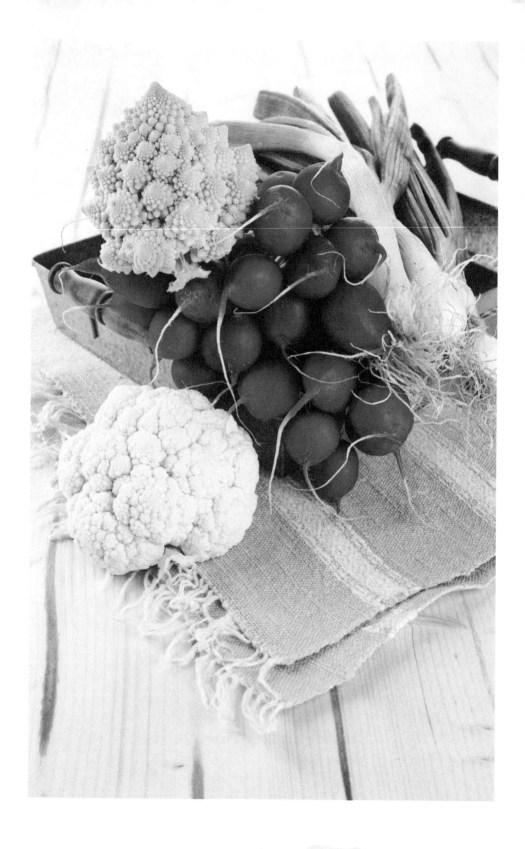

What Is the DASH Diet?

How the DASH Diet Came to Life

In August 1993, a group of fifty researchers—including several doctors and dietitians from top medical institutions, such as Harvard Medical School, Duke University School of Medicine, and Johns Hopkins Medical Center—came together to design an eating program that would reliably reduce blood pressure. Twelve months later, their study was underway, and by its end, 459 volunteers were enjoying the benefits the DASH diet provides. Not only did the study's participants gain the advantage of decreased blood pressure, many of them lost weight, even though weight loss wasn't the study's original goal.

Over the past twenty years, what began as a dietary approach for reducing hypertension (high blood pressure) has become a respected plan for reliable weight loss; in fact, in their 2013 diet rankings *U.S. News & World Report* ranked the DASH diet number one in the "Best Diets Overall" category, comparing it against twenty-eight other diets, including popular plans such as the South Beach Diet, Jenny Craig, and Weight Watchers.

To an outside observer, someone following the DASH diet may not appear to be on a diet at all. That's because DASH is not strictly structured as so many weight-loss regimens are; instead, it is a tool anyone can use to generate a healthier lifestyle while enjoying a varied yet balanced combination of delicious foods. Followers of the plan can take comfort in the fact that their new choices are backed by extensive research and scientific evidence as well as endorsed by some of the world's most respected health care organizations, including National Institutes of Health, the American Dietetic Association, the American Heart Association, and the U.S. Department of Health and Human Services.

Dietary Approaches to Stop Hypertension

DASH is an acronym for "Dietary Approaches to Stop Hypertension." Besides having been designed by nutritional and medical scientists, the original research behind the plan was funded by the National Institutes of Health. This means that DASH was not crafted by a corporation intent on pushing products and meeting profit margin goals. Nor is DASH a fad diet. Anyone—no matter what foods he or she prefers—will find the diet's guidelines simple, even second nature to follow. You don't have to seek out specific brands or whip up strange concoctions; instead, all you have to do is focus on eating real foods in sensible quantities.

The DASH meal plan emphasizes vegetables, fruits, and low-fat dairy products. It includes plenty of whole grains along with seafood, poultry, and nuts. Many of these foods contain high levels of potassium, calcium, or magnesium and are recommended not only for their nutrition but also because they aid in reducing blood pressure.

What's on Your Plate?

Based on 2,000 calories per day, the DASH diet includes:

- 7 to 8 servings of grain daily, with at least 3 whole-grain foods consumed each day

- 4 to 5 servings of fruits daily

- 4 to 5 servings of vegetables daily

- 2 to 3 servings of low-fat or nonfat dairy foods daily

- 2 or fewer servings of lean meat, poultry, fish, or seafood daily

- Limited (less than 2) servings of fats and sweets (combined) daily

- 4 to 5 servings of nuts, seeds, or legumes weekly

- No more than 2 alcoholic beverages for men; no more than 1 alcoholic beverage for women

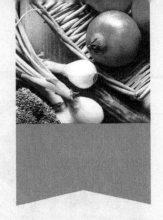

PART TWO

DASH Diet Health Plan

Chapter Three DASH Diet for High Blood Pressure / Hypertension

Chapter Four DASH Diet for Weight Loss

Chapter Five DASH Diet for Optimal Health

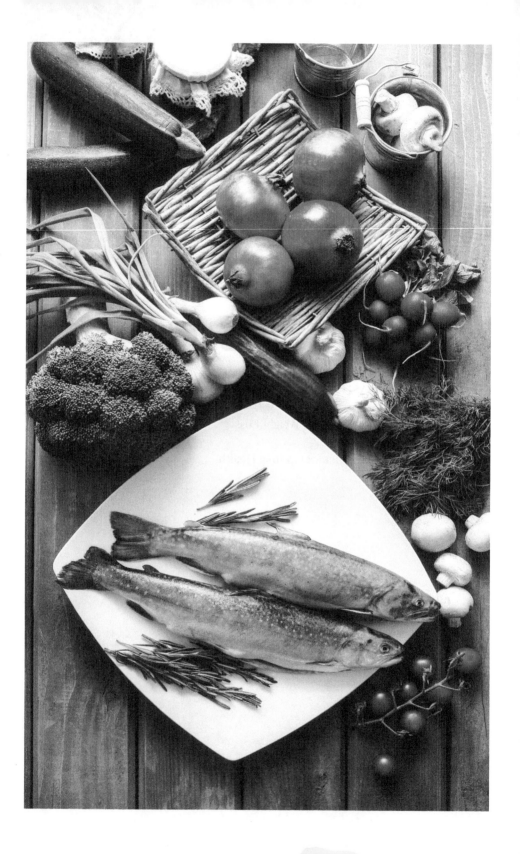

DASH Diet for High Blood Pressure / Hypertension

How Reducing Sodium Alleviates High Blood Pressure

For some people in certain at-risk categories, including those who are obese, men and women over age sixty, and those of African American descent, a high-sodium diet contributes to high blood pressure. This happens because sodium causes the body to retain excess fluid, which in turn makes it harder for the heart to push blood through arteries and blood vessels. The extra effort not only taxes the heart, it increases pressure on the arteries.

When sodium intake is reduced, as it is in the DASH diet, excess fluid is eliminated, allowing the heart to propel blood through the body with much less effort. As a result, blood pressure is typically decreased.

Understanding Hypertension

Though most people are aware that high blood pressure is a health problem, many are unsure what the term actually means. Blood pressure is a measure of the force that blood exerts against arterial walls. In hypertension, blood pushes against those arterial walls with excess force. If you were to measure your blood pressure over the course of a day, you'd find that it goes up and down—but when it remains elevated over time, hypertension is usually the diagnosis. High blood pressure endangers the body by forcing the heart to work harder than it should, causing damage to arteries in the resulting high-pressure blood flow. There are typically no signs or symptoms that high blood pressure is approaching, and once it occurs, it often lasts for the rest of the sufferer's life.

Know Your Numbers

Hypertension is increased pressure in the arteries that carry blood from the heart to all the tissues and organs of the body. An elevation in either the systolic or diastolic blood pressure increases the risk of developing heart disease, kidney disease, hardening of the arteries, eye damage, and stroke.

The next time you have your blood pressure checked, use the following numbers to see where you fall.

The systolic blood pressure is the upper number in a blood pressure reading, measured in millimeters of mercury:

- Normal = Less than 120
- Prehypertension = 120–139
- Hypertension = 140 or higher

The diastolic blood pressure is the lower number, measured in millimeters of mercury:

- Normal = Less than 80
- Prehypertension = 80–89
- Hypertension = 90 or higher

If you're above the normal range, following the DASH diet to make better food choices and get your sodium intake under control will result in the satisfaction of watching these numbers go down, right along with that one on the scale.

In America alone, one in four adults—more than fifty million people—suffer from hypertension. Possible risk factors include:

- Aging
- Being overweight or obese
- Chronic kidney disorders
- Excessive alcohol consumption (more than 1 to 2 drinks daily)
- Excessive salt intake
- Family history of hypertension
- Genetic makeup

- Physical inactivity

- Stress

- Thyroid and adrenal disorders

Though health experts are aware that people with high blood pressure share at least some of these traits, the exact underlying cause of hypertension is unknown. However, it's no secret that the condition tends to run in families and that it is historically more likely to affect men than women. In the United States, African Americans are twice as likely as Caucasians to suffer from high blood pressure, though that gap starts to narrow at age forty-four. After the age of sixty-five, it widens again, at which point African American women have the highest rate of hypertension.

Regardless of your background, if you have high blood pressure, it is certain to have an adverse effect on your overall health, particularly if it continues over time. Hypertension is linked to cardiovascular diseases and to stroke—both of which are leading causes of disability and premature death.

While it is possible in many cases to control blood pressure with prescription drugs, these pharmaceuticals, which come with potentially dangerous side effects, are not the only solution. In fact, they do not address hypertension itself; they merely treat the symptoms. Dietary and lifestyle changes are the surest way to reduce or eliminate high blood pressure for good, either lessening the need for pharmaceuticals or completely eliminating it.

You might imagine that adopting a dietary approach to reversing or preventing hypertension would take a while to yield results; however, many people who have faithfully followed the DASH diet have been able to decrease their blood pressure in as little as two weeks—even without the use of medications.

Many doctors prescribe the DASH diet in addition to high blood pressure medication in order to provide patients with a dual-pronged approach to managing hypertension. To make treatment even more effective, patients are often advised to begin an exercise regimen. Walking for as little as thirty minutes three times per week can help bring blood pressure down. When the DASH diet is combined with exercise, people who are prescribed blood pressure medication are often able to taper off and eventually stop taking it altogether.

An Emphasis on Whole, Healthful Foods

The DASH diet is far from extreme. It simply emphasizes vegetables, fruits, whole grains, and legumes, along with low-fat dairy, nuts, and moderate amounts of fish and poultry.

Although you can enjoy food of any type and still follow the DASH diet, there are several foods that can contribute to increased high blood pressure. It's recommended that these items either be consumed in very small amounts or not at all. These foods include:

- Products that are high in saturated fat, such as fast foods, fatty meats, full-fat dairy products, egg yolks, and processed meats.

- Foods high in cholesterol, such as fatty or marbled meats, full-fat dairy products, egg yolks, fast foods, canned fish packed in oil, and processed meats.

- Foods containing trans fats, which doctors consider to be the worst type of fat in the modern diet, such as anything containing hydrogenated or partially hydrogenated vegetable oil and fried foods, like French fries, onion rings, and donuts.

- Sweets, such as candies, cakes, and other desserts, as well as other foods that are high in sugar, particularly hidden sugars. For example, many salad dressings, sauces, and processed foods, such as spaghetti sauce and pizza, contain a surprising amount of sugar.

Consuming too much sugar, particularly fructose, can cause your blood pressure to increase. Fructose is a key ingredient in high-fructose corn syrup (HFCS), which is present in many products, ranging from non-diet soda to ketchup. A daily habit of drinking 30 ounces of soda made with HFCS or consuming the same amount of fructose from other sources can increase your risk of hypertension by at least 30 percent, whether you consume a low-sodium diet or not. While HFCS is the most dangerous type of sugar, other added sugars can increase your risk of hypertension as well. When using the DASH diet for hypertension, consume no more than five sweet treats per week, and be on the lookout for added sugar in everything from salad dressing to crackers.

The DASH diet is not a reduced-calorie diet. Instead, it is a well-balanced eating plan based on an intake of 2,000 calories per day. If you are tall or very active, you may need more calories to maintain a healthful body weight while reducing your blood pressure; if you are aging, sedentary, or short, or if you have a very small frame, you may require fewer calories. If you are overweight, you can follow the DASH diet for weight loss while working to eliminate hypertension.

Focusing on reducing sodium, eliminating unhealthful fats, and cutting back on sweets may sound like a difficult task, but since only small amounts of sodium occur naturally in whole, unprocessed foods, which are generally much higher in fiber than processed versions, the options are almost endless.

SMART SODIUM CHOICES: WHERE'S THE SODIUM?

Food Group	Average Sodium Content
Grains	
Unsalted cooked pasta, rice, or hot whole-grain cereal, ½ cup	0–5 mg
Dry cereal, 1 cup	100–360 mg
Bread, 1 slice	110–175 mg
Vegetables	
Fresh or frozen varieties, no salt added, ½ cup	0–70 mg
Canned or frozen, with added sauce, ½ cup	140–460 mg
Canned tomato juice, ¾ cup	820 mg
Fruit	
Fresh, frozen, or canned, ½ cup	0–5 mg
Dairy	
Low-fat or fat-free milk, 1 cup	120 mg
Yogurt, 8 ounces	160 mg
Natural cheeses, 1½ ounces	110–450 mg
Processed cheeses, 1½ ounces	600 mg
Nuts and Legumes	
Peanuts, unsalted, 3 ounces	0–5 mg
Beans, frozen or dried, no salt added, ½ cup	0–5 mg
Peanuts, salted, 3 ounces	120 mg
Beans, canned, ½ cup	400 mg
Fish, Poultry, and Meat	
Fresh fish, poultry, or meat, 3 ounces	30–90 mg
Canned tuna packed in water, no salt added, 3 ounces	35–45 mg
Canned tuna packed in water, with salt, 3 ounces	250–350 mg
Reduced-sodium turkey deli slices, 2 ounces	440 mg
Roasted ham, 3 ounces	1,020 mg

Source: U.S. Department of Health and Human Services

CHAPTER FOUR

DASH Diet for Weight Loss

The DASH diet, though created for the purpose of reversing hypertension, is also a satisfying, nutritious eating plan that has been proved to lead to lasting weight loss. Better yet, it's a well-balanced, sustainable diet that can be followed for a lifetime in order to maintain a healthful weight after excess pounds have been shed.

When using the DASH diet for weight loss, the focus remains on whole, healthful foods; however, weight loss is accelerated when the bulk of each day's intake is made up of high-fiber, low-calorie foods that are slow to digest. These foods have also been linked to a lower incidence of diabetes, cancer, heart disease, and even osteoporosis.

With many weight-loss diets, particularly extreme diets that eliminate certain food groups altogether, the exact opposite is true; it's impossible to stick with many of these plans for long, and as a result, any weight discarded has a tendency to creep back on once the diet comes to an end. Since foods recommended by the creators of the DASH diet are nutritious, delicious, and easy to obtain, many people find this plan to be one they can realistically follow—and enjoy—for the rest of their lives.

The DASH diet for weight loss includes so many fruits and vegetables that you may wonder how you'll be able to eat the required servings during the course of a day. Dividing your daily intake into four to six mini meals instead of three large ones can make eating these high-volume foods easier. In addition, this approach will help you feel full all day, making unhealthful foods much less tempting.

Good preparation is essential to making any new endeavor successful. You need to know that you have the right tools and supplies—and that your goals are realistic—before you get started.

Date:

Weight:

Neck:

Waist Women **:**

Hips Women **:**

Abdomen Men **:**

Body Fat %:

BMR: calories

DCR:

What Is Your Body Mass Index?

The first thing you need to do is establish your health and fitness goals. Most people rely on the bathroom scale to tell them how much weight they need to lose, but that's really not the most accurate measurement.

Start by determining your body mass index (BMI). This index approximates the percentage of your body weight that is fat. You can get your body fat calculated by professionals or purchase a body fat measurement kit; alternately, you can get a fairly accurate measurement of your BMI with a measuring tape and an online calculator.

Next, measure your weight. To do this, you'll need to weigh yourself first thing in the morning, after urinating and before eating or drinking. Wear only your underwear or nothing at all. Record your weight in the appropriate blank on the BMI Assessment Form.

Next, you'll need to gather some measurements to use in calculating your BMI.

For men, you'll measure your neck and abdomen circumference. Be sure the measuring tape keeps in contact with your skin without pulling it too tightly. To measure your abdomen, wrap the measuring tape around your body at a point just below your belly button.

For women, you'll measure the circumference of your neck, waist, and hips. Measure your waist at the slimmest point of your torso and measure your hips just below the hip bones; the measuring tape should cross the top portion of your buttocks. As you take these measurements, you can write them down on the BMI Assessment Form.

Once you have your measurements, you can calculate your BMI using one of the many free calculators that are available online, http://www.nhlbi.nih.gov/ or http://www.linear-software.com/online.html.

If you are using the calculator in the link, take the following steps to calculate your BMI are:

- Find the section that pertains to your gender.

- Enter your age and weight.

- Enter your measurements in the "Tape Measurement Method" column.

- Click the "Calculate" button.

- Scroll down to see your results.

Once you have determined your body fat percentage using an online calculator, enter the value on the "Body Fat %" line of the BMI Assessment Form.

With an understanding of your body fat percentage, you can begin understanding your current state of health and have a point of comparison after you have started following the DASH diet. While you can weigh yourself along the way and celebrate pounds lost, recalculating your BMI is often a more efficient way to track your progress.

If you follow both the DASH diet and the DASH to Fitness workout plan, you'll likely be gaining lean muscle mass as you lose fat. In this situation, a scale can't tell the difference between muscle weight and fat weight; lean muscle weighs more than fat but is more compact than fat tissue. As a result, the scale may say you've gained weight, but you are likely to see an improvement in your BMI. To see an example of this improvement in action, you can return to the BMI calculator you used for your initial calculation and reduce your measurements by several inches (just one or two inches at the neck, and a few to several inches at the waist, abdomen, or hips). This will show what your BMI would be given those hypothetical measurements.

What Is Your Basal Metabolic Rate?

Once you have an understanding of your BMI, it is important to calculate the number of calories that your body requires to maintain your current weight. This calculation will help you understand the number of calories you should consume in order to lose weight at a safe and comfortable pace.

To perform this calculation, first you need to calculate your basal metabolic rate (BMR). The BMR formula takes your height, weight, age, and gender into account in its calculation. This method is likely to be more accurate than calculating your calorie needs based solely on body weight. Since leaner bodies burn more calories than less lean ones, this method will be accurate unless you are very muscular or very obese. If you're very fit and muscular, you may need to add more calories, and if you're very overweight you may need to deduct them. Trial and error will help you make these types of adjustments as you progress in your diet.

The following formula will calculate your BMR:

- **For Women**: BMR = 655 + (4.35 × weight in pounds) + (4.7 × height in inches) – (4.7 × age in years)

- **For Men**: BMR = 66 + (6.23 × weight in pounds) + (12.7 × height in inches) – (6.8 × age in year)

Calculate your BMR and record it in on the BMI Assessment Form.

What Are Your Daily Calorie Requirements?

To determine your daily calorie requirements (DCR) you'll need to factor in your activity level. To do this, we use what is known as the Harris Benedict Equation.

To determine your total daily calorie needs, multiply your BMR by the appropriate activity factor, as follows:

- If you are sedentary (little or no exercise):
  DCR = BMR × 1.2

- If you are lightly active (exercise 1–3 days a week):
  DCR = BMR × 1.375

- If you are moderately active (exercise 3–5 days a week):
  DCR = BMR × 1.55

- If you are very active (exercise 6–7 days a week):
  DCR = BMR × 1.725

- If you are extra active (exercise daily and have a physical job or are training):
  DCR = BMR × 1.9

Calculate your DCR and record it on the BMI Assessment Form.

Once you know the number of calories needed to maintain your weight, you can easily calculate the number of calories you need to eat in order to gain or lose weight.

One pound equals 3,500 calories, so to lose one pound a week you would deduct 500 calories from your total DCR (not your BMR). To lose two pounds a week, you would need to deduct 1,000 calories per day.

For people whose DCR is low, trying to lose weight solely by cutting calories may be impractical and unsustainable. It's healthful to combine increased activity and decreased calorie intake, but this is especially true for those who already have a low calorie requirement.

You can start out using the caloric requirements for your present activity level, minus 500–1,000 calories per day. In two weeks, if you're staying on schedule with your DASH to Fitness plan, recalculate your DCR using the appropriate new activity level. This will ensure that you're getting enough nutrition yet still staying on track for your weight loss.

The DASH Diet Health Plan does not recommend cutting calories below 1,500 per day for women and 1,800 per day for men.

Exercise and the DASH Diet

One of the easiest ways to identify a fad diet that likely won't work long-term is to listen for the words "no exercise required." Exercise, even in small amounts, is essential for everyone—not just for weight loss but also for good physical and mental health. One of the most amazing things about the human body is its ability to regain flexibility and stamina, even in people who have been living sedentary lives for many years or even decades.

While there are diets that call for intense exercise on a regular basis, the DASH diet takes a less stringent approach. Only about 15 percent of Americans exercise daily. With this figure in mind, the diet's developers recommend that participants who are out of shape simply begin walking a few times per week, for a few minutes at a time. Eventually, even the least fit people can work their way up to high levels of activity as their bodies become accustomed to regular exercise.

Not only is walking considered to be one of the safest low-impact exercises, it is also economical. All you need are comfortable clothes, supportive walking shoes, and perhaps your favorite music or audiobook to keep you company. Best of all, you can walk just about anywhere—your neighborhood, a local mall, a park, or even inside an airport while awaiting a flight.

If you are in poor physical condition, be sure to talk with your doctor about starting a fitness routine, even if it is just walking. Once your condition improves and the weight starts to come off, you'll likely discover yourself feeling increasingly motivated, plus you'll be able to walk faster. The faster you're able to walk, the more calories you'll burn, the better you'll condition your cardiovascular system, and the healthier you will feel and look.

There is another reason to stick with regular exercise while following the DASH diet, whether your aim is weight loss, reversing hypertension, or simply overall health: The combination of moderate exercise and sustainable diet has been shown to improve mental activity by an average of 30 percent as compared with overweight adults who did not modify their diets or engage in exercise. Researchers believe that these simple lifestyle modifications have significant implications for potentially slowing or even reversing cognitive defects that can occur with age, including dementia and Alzheimer's disease.

The four-month study, which was published in *Hypertension: Journal of the American Heart Association*, focused on 124 overweight adults who were divided into three groups. The first group followed the DASH diet and participated in thirty minutes of aerobic exercise three times each week. The second group followed the DASH diet but did not exercise, and the third group did not exercise or diet.

At the end of the study, not only did mental activity improve for the first group, their lifestyle changes showed improved cardiovascular fitness, reduced systolic blood pressure by an average of sixteen points, reduced diastolic blood pressure by an average of ten points, and an average weight loss of nineteen pounds.

Exercising with a friend can help you better adhere to your routine. Find a friend or family member who would like to make exercise a regular part of his or her life, then set a schedule and stick to it. This strategy works well because exercise partners are often reluctant to let one another down; plus socializing while working out is a fun way to connect and improve social bonds.

DASH Diet for Optimal Health

Medicine Be Thy Food

More than two thousand years ago, the Greek physician Hippocrates gave the following advice: "Let food be thy medicine and medicine be thy food." We could do worse than follow his counsel today. With the right diet, you'll find that it is much easier to maintain good health—and with physical well-being, comes the ability to enjoy a naturally high energy level and a positive frame of mind.

The DASH diet is perfect for anyone looking to improve overall health. If your goals include living longer, maintaining a healthful weight, and reducing your risk of suffering from heart disease, stroke, and other debilitating health problems, this method of eating will help you meet all of those goals.

Cardiovascular Benefits

Rigorous studies have shown that the DASH diet's ability to lower blood pressure makes it ideal for maintaining heart health. Cardiovascular benefits include:

- Reducing the risk of hypertension, even if you are in an at-risk category

- Maintaining healthful cholesterol levels and, in turn, preventing hardened arteries

- Keeping triglycerides low to reduce the overall risk of heart disease

Because of its emphasis on plant-based foods and keeping excess salt, sugar, and saturated fat off your plate, the DASH diet reflects the health care community's definition of the ideal diet for heart health.

When plant-based foods make up the bulk of an individual's diet, the heart greatly benefits. Studies have shown that people who eat an abundance of fruits, vegetables, legumes, nuts, and other plant-based foods have a 20 percent lower risk of developing heart disease and a 27 percent reduced risk of dying of cardiovascular disease. Further research shows that each ten-gram increase in daily fiber intake is associated with an additional 27 percent reduction in risk of death from heart disease.

Conformity with Accepted Dietary Intake Guidelines

When you follow the DASH diet, you will be well within federal dietary intake guidelines—something that cannot be said about many other eating plans, and certainly not the standard American diet. When comparing methods of eating for optimal health, be sure to consider:

- Calcium—Essential for building and maintaining bones and teeth, calcium is also critical to proper muscle and blood vessel function. The current recommended daily intake is between 1,000 and 1,300 mg. The DASH diet, with its focus on low-fat dairy and calcium-rich vegetables and fruits, provides more than enough.

- Carbohydrates—The DASH diet contains all the whole, healthful carbohydrates required for sustained energy—they're absorbed slowly, so you feel full longer and your blood sugar level remains stable.

- Fat content—Current guidelines recommend that daily intake consist of between 20 and 35 percent healthful fat; with the DASH diet, you'll get just the right amount.

- Fiber—Current guidelines call for adults to consume at least 22 grams of fiber daily. The DASH diet provides you with all the fiber you need.

- Potassium—Potassium plays a special role in countering salt's ability to raise blood pressure; it also decreases bone loss and reduces the risk of kidney stones. Most Americans consume less than the recommended 4,700 mg per day; however, the DASH diet provides almost 5,000 mg and is one of the few plans that does so.

- Salt—While the recommended daily maximum sodium intake is 2,300 mg, if you are age fifty-one or older, of African American descent, or if you have diabetes, chronic kidney disease, or hypertension, it's best to consume no more than about 1,500 mg per day. There are DASH diet plans designed for both of these maximum sodium levels.

- Saturated fat content—No more than 10 percent of your daily calorie intake should come from saturated fat; with the DASH diet, it is easy to stay out of the danger zone.

- Vitamin B_{12}—Adults need at least 2.4 micrograms of vitamin B_{12}, which plays a vital role in healthful metabolism at a cellular level. You'll get plenty while following the DASH plan.

Many people who begin a plant-based diet worry about feeling less than satisfied after a meal. When it comes to producing feelings of fullness, the DASH diet is one of the best out there: Fruits, vegetables, and whole grains do a fantastic job of keeping you sated, as do the nuts, lean proteins, and low-fat dairy options you can enjoy while following this plan.

Recommendations for Using the DASH Diet for Optimal Health

One of the reasons people enjoy and stick with the DASH diet is that nothing is really forbidden. No matter which foods are your favorites, you can work them into your eating plan, either by enjoying a small amount every now and then, or better yet, by learning to make treasured recipes healthier. If you are a vegetarian or vegan, or if you'd like to reduce your cholesterol and triglyceride levels even further, it's very easy to substitute plant-based products such as tofu, tempeh, seitan, vegan cheeses, soy milk, and nut milks for those you'd rather not consume.

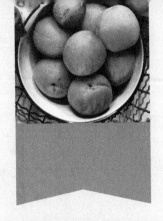

PART **THREE**

Transitioning to the DASH Diet

Chapter Six Tips for Planning Your DASH Diet

Chapter Seven DASH Diet Food Groups

Chapter Eight Ten Steps for Success

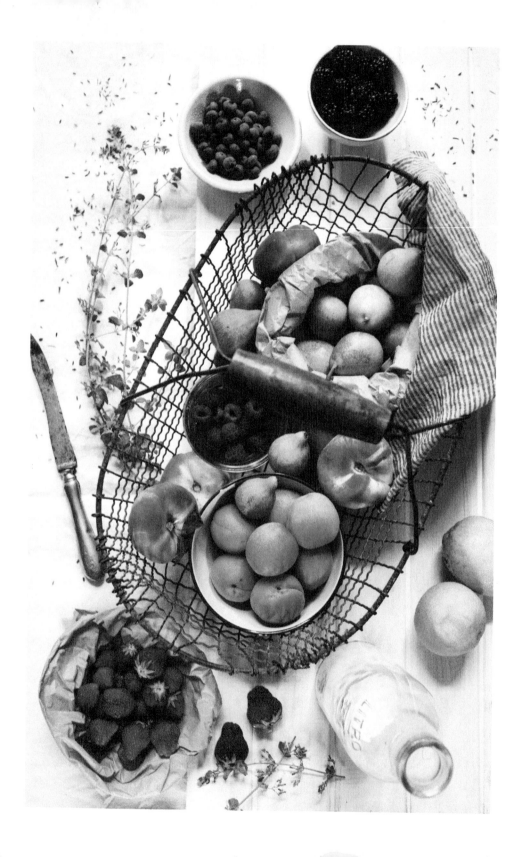

Tips for Planning Your DASH Diet

How to Get Started

While it might be tempting to skip the planning stage and simply dive right into dieting, it is essential to devote some thought to how incorporating DASH into your meal plan will affect every facet of your life. Smart planning is one of the best ways to ensure that you are successful with the DASH diet. Normally, you might think to plan your meals only on special occasions—such as holidays, birthdays, and other social gatherings—but changing this way of thinking and creating both long-term and short-term eating plans will decrease the likelihood that you'll fall back into old, destructive eating patterns. You wouldn't venture out on a long road trip without a map or GPS system, so why start a journey as important as this without some forethought?

When you eat is just as important as *what* you eat. Planning mealtimes and snack times helps ensure that your body stays fueled and does not enter calorie-conservation mode. Start your day with a sizable breakfast, enjoy a snack about two hours before lunch, and have another snack about two hours prior to dinner. It may seem counter-intuitive at first, but try to make dinner the smallest meal of the day rather than the largest, and make a habit of not eating for at least three hours before bedtime. This way, your body uses the food you eat rather than storing it as fat.

What's Your Motivation?

To be successful with the DASH diet, it's vital that you understand why you want to be healthier or weigh less. Before getting started, spend some time thinking about your reasons for beginning this program as well as considering your commitment level:

- Is my motivation coming from an outside source or am I self-motivated?

- Am I ready for this plan?

- What if setbacks occur? How will I deal with them?

- Am I committed to making the necessary changes?

- Is my family committed to supporting me? If not, why not?

Determine Your Weight and BMI

Before beginning the DASH diet, it's important that you know your weight and your body mass index (BMI). If you haven't stepped on a scale in years, now is the time to do it. You may also want to measure your waist, hips, chest, thighs, upper arms, and calves before beginning the plan, as these measurements will serve as another method for tracking success.

Decide on a system for recording your statistics, or use a free online weight tracker or smartphone app before taking your first set of measurements.

Begin by checking your weight, and plan to weigh yourself once each week at about the same time on a set day; for example, you can choose to weigh yourself every Wednesday morning before breakfast.

After you get your starting weight, use the table on the right to determine your BMI. Round your weight up or down to the nearest 10 pounds; then look at the point where that number intersects with your height. For example, if you weigh 200 pounds and you are five feet six inches tall, your BMI is 32.

Next, interpret your BMI:

- Under 18.5: Underweight

- 18.5–24: Normal weight

- 24–29: Overweight

- 30 or higher: Obese

If you fall in the obese category, determine what your level of obesity is:

- 30–34: Class I obesity

- 35–39: Class II obesity

- 40 or higher: Class III obesity

Weight

Height	100	110	120	130	140	150	160	170	180	190	200	210	220	230	240	250
5'0"	20	21	23	25	27	29	31	33	35	37	39	41	43	45	47	49
5'1"	19	21	23	25	26	28	30	32	34	36	38	40	42	43	45	47
5'2"	18	20	22	24	26	27	29	31	33	35	37	38	40	42	44	46
5'3"	18	19	21	23	25	27	28	30	32	34	35	37	39	41	43	44
5'4"	17	19	21	22	24	26	27	29	31	33	34	36	38	39	41	43
5'5"	17	18	20	22	23	25	27	28	30	32	33	35	37	38	40	42
5'6"	16	18	19	21	23	24	26	27	29	31	32	34	36	37	39	40
5'7"	16	17	19	20	22	23	25	27	28	30	31	33	34	36	38	39
5'8"	15	17	18	20	21	23	24	26	27	29	30	32	33	35	36	38
5'9"	15	16	18	19	21	22	24	25	27	28	30	31	32	34	35	37
5'10"	14	16	17	19	20	22	23	24	26	27	29	30	32	33	34	36
5'11"	14	15	17	18	20	21	22	24	25	26	27	28	30	32	33	35
6'0"	14	15	16	18	19	20	22	23	24	26	27	28	30	31	33	34
6'1"	13	15	16	17	18	20	21	22	24	25	26	28	29	30	32	33
6'2"	13	14	15	17	18	19	21	22	23	24	26	27	28	30	31	32
6'3"	12	14	15	16	17	19	20	21	22	24	25	26	27	29	30	31
6'4"	12	13	15	16	17	18	19	21	22	23	24	26	27	28	29	30

Source: http://www.health.harvard.edu/topic/BMI-Calculator

No matter what your BMI, and no matter how alarmed you may feel at the numbers that show up on the scale, it's important that you view these figures as a starting point rather than as cause for discouragement. You might find it helpful to remind yourself that you are just one of the nearly 50 percent of Americans who are overweight.

Whatever you do, don't fall into the trap of berating yourself for what you see in front of you. Yes, certain actions or inaction did contribute to those numbers, but it is important to focus on where you are going rather than to beat yourself up about where you've been.

Treat Yourself to a Physical

If you haven't had a physical recently, get one as soon as you can. Obtaining your weight and determining your BMI are not difficult to do on your own; however, it's equally important that you find out your cholesterol levels and blood pressure before you begin to follow the DASH diet. It's also an excellent idea to discuss your dietary plans with your doctor before beginning. He or she will probably offer encouragement and point you toward additional resources that can increase your chances of success. As you make progress on the plan, you may want to return to your health care provider for wellness checks; seeing improvements and tracking those numbers along with your weight, BMI, and body measurements will help spur you toward your final goals and ultimately toward maintaining good health in the future.

Set Attainable Goals

You may have a long-term goal for weight loss or for better health; perhaps you want to reduce your cholesterol by a certain number of points, or maybe you've set your heart on fitting into a certain size of clothing. If you don't have far to go to meet those goals, setting a single milestone might work well for you.

If you need to lose more than 10 pounds, or if you are in crisis where blood pressure, cholesterol, or other measurable markers of physical health are concerned, break your larger goal or goals into smaller ones that will be easy for you to achieve. As you meet one goal after another, your confidence in your ability to succeed will improve, and you will gain momentum.

Either way, it's important that you pick specific, measurable goals ahead of time that can serve as benchmarks of your success. For example, if you set a generalized goal of losing weight and becoming healthier, you might see only a moderate amount of improvement. If, on the other hand, you focus on specific targets, such as committing to lose 1 pound per week or a specified number of pounds over the course of a month, you'll find it easier to stay motivated, particularly when the goals you set for yourself are within easy reach. It is incredibly satisfying to keep track of each milestone and strive to complete the next one, and when you do this, you are likely to see significant results and improve your health more rapidly.

Tips for Reducing Calorie Intake

The following are some ideas for consuming fewer calories while following the DASH diet:

- Eat a meatless meal at least once a week.
- Try baked kale leaves or a handful of dried fruit for a snack instead of potato chips.
- Treat yourself with half a cup of low-fat frozen yogurt instead of ice cream.
- Choose fat-free or low-fat condiments and dairy products.
- Reduce vegetable oil, margarine, mayonnaise, and salad dressings by half.
- Always read food labels for fat content in packaged foods.
- Cut back on all foods with added sugar.
- Eat fruits canned in their own juice or in water.
- Snack on unbuttered, unsalted popcorn or rice cakes.
- Drink water or club soda with a wedge of lemon or lime.

Eliminate Undesirable Foods and Sources of Temptation

After you have calculated your weight and BMI, along with any other measurements, it's time to eliminate sources of temptation. The best place to begin is in your home pantry and refrigerator.

Start by reading labels. Foods that contain a high percentage of sodium, high-fructose corn syrup, and/or hydrogenated fats or partially hydrogenated fats should be eliminated immediately, including:

- Potato chips, pretzels, and other salty snack foods

- Packaged deli meats

- Dry cereals with sugar, artificial coloring, and other additives

- Canned goods, including vegetables and beans, unless they are low-sodium

- Frozen pizzas, jarred sauces, prepackaged meals, and other highly processed items

- Candy, ice cream, cookies, and other sweets

- High-fat cheeses and whole milk

Natural Is Heart Healthful

Only a very small amount of our daily sodium intake comes from the saltshaker on our table. And food in its natural state contains very little sodium; it's processed food that is the primary enabler of our sodium addiction. The sad truth is that the more we "mess around" with our food—filling it with additives, wrapping it in plastic, and generally making it unrecognizable from its original state—the less good for us it becomes. This is why it is so important to eat natural, whole foods whenever possible.

For example, the DASH diet emphasizes the potassium content of whole foods, especially that of fruits and vegetables, which helps keep blood pressure levels healthful. Some dairy products and fish are also rich sources of natural potassium. However, fruits and vegetables are rich in a particular form of potassium that positively influences acid-base metabolism. It is believed this form of potassium helps reduce the risk of kidney stones and bone loss.

While you might think that canned vegetables are a healthful substitute for fresh ones, the exact opposite can be true: canned vegetables are sometimes laden with preservatives, and they often contain added salt. A single serving of canned cream-style corn, for example, may contain as much as 730 milligrams of sodium per cup. Choose low-sodium canned vegetables or frozen vegetables without sauces instead, and eat as much fresh produce as possible.

It can be difficult to part with old favorites, and many people are tempted to finish unhealthful items rather than waste them. Keep in mind, though, that all these foods are ultimately going to end up as waste—whether they go through your body or not. Why eat them when you could make healthful choices instead?

If your budget demands that you slowly phase out various items, do so, and watch your portions carefully. If you're considering keeping certain items on hand because they are family favorites, keep in mind that what isn't ideal for your own diet isn't the best for your family's, either. It might take a little effort to find or make replacements, but the payoff in terms of your and your loved ones' health is worth the effort.

Next, think about when and where you typically consume unhealthful food items. If you have a tendency to hit the office vending machine when you feel hungry, bored, or stressed at work, plant some nutritious snacks within easy reach of your desk. Packages of unsalted or lightly salted nuts, dried fruit, and even certain energy bars or meal-replacement bars can prevent a binge.

Canned soups and jarred pasta sauces are convenient, but they often contain high levels of sodium as well as added sugar. For example, a single cup of canned chicken noodle soup typically contains about 744 milligrams of sodium, while a serving of condensed tomato soup contains about 480 milligrams of sodium and 12 grams of sugar. Some food manufacturers are working hard to provide their customers with healthier choices, so look for low-sodium and reduced-sugar varieties.

Perhaps you regularly grab quick lunches out or stop by your favorite fast-food joint while running errands. To curb this bad habit, store a few healthful snacks in your glove compartment so you have something to reach for when hunger strikes. If simply seeing a particular fast-food sign is a trigger for unhealthful cravings, take a different route that will limit exposure to temptation.

Gain Portion-Control Awareness

Many people are shocked when they discover just how much larger today's portion sizes are than they were just twenty years ago. It's not your fault that you are eating larger portions; you have been trained to expect them. During the 1990s, the size of the average dinner plate grew from 10 inches across to 12 inches across; at the same time, bowls and cups also expanded.

That's not all; portions at restaurants have become massively oversized as well. In fact, current portion sizes at fast-food chains are, on average, two to five times larger than they were when those restaurants were first established. McDonald's first hamburger weighed in at a reasonable 1.6 ounces. Today, you can get a Double Quarter Pounder with cheese, which features two beef patties weighing 4 ounces apiece before cooking—that's half a pound of meat! This monstrous sandwich contains 750 calories, 43 grams of fat, and 1,280 milligrams of sodium.

This is just one example; menu items at other restaurants have ballooned to an outrageous size as well. The good news is that if you're planning to eat at a restaurant or enjoy a snack away from home, you can usually find solid information concerning calorie count, fat, and sodium online. Many states now require restaurants to display calorie information on menus. Knowing what is hiding in your food can be very helpful when it comes time to decide what to eat and what to leave behind.

POPULAR FOODS TWENTY YEARS AGO VERSUS TODAY

Food	Twenty Years Ago	Today
Bagel	3-inch diameter, 140 calories	6-inch diameter, 350 calories or more
Coffee	8-ounce cup with cream and sugar, 45 calories	16 ounces with cream and sugar, 350 calories or more
Fast-food cheeseburger	333 calories	590 calories
Movie popcorn	5 cups, 270 calories	1 large tub, 630 calories
Pizza	2 slices, 500 calories	2 slices, 850 calories
Soda	6.5-ounce bottle, 82 calories	20-ounce bottle, 250 calories

Source: National Heart, Lung, and Blood Institute

CHAPTER SEVEN

DASH Diet Food Groups

What to Eat: Recommended DASH Diet Foods

No matter which version of the DASH diet you decide to follow, you'll find that both plans call for the same basic types of food. The daily number of servings of each type will vary depending on your caloric needs.

Grains

Focus on eating whole grains. Cereals, brown rice, whole-grain pasta, whole-grain bread, and other grains like barley, quinoa, and amaranth, contain fiber, healthful carbohydrates, and a wide range of vitamins and minerals that are essential to good health.

Since processed grain products are lower in both fiber and protein, and because they are digested much more rapidly than whole grains are, they should be avoided. Processed grains include white rice, most commercial breads and crackers, many cereals, and anything else made with refined flour, including baked goods.

The most healthful grains for you tend to be the simplest. Oatmeal, particularly the steel-cut or "Irish" variety, contains both soluble and insoluble fiber, keeping you feeling satisfied longer and helping to sweep lipids from your circulatory system. If preparing whole grains seems troublesome and time-consuming, consider making a large batch and placing individual portions in microwaveable containers for later convenience.

Vegetables

The best vegetables for losing weight with the DASH diet include fresh leafy greens; cruciferous vegetables, such as broccoli and cauliflower; colorful favorites like carrots, tomatoes, and bell peppers; and many others, including green beans, sweet peas, and corn. Beans and peas are also legumes, and are higher in calories, fiber, and protein than are many other vegetables.

There are only a few types of vegetables that ought to be consumed with care. Potatoes need to be limited, as they are rapidly transformed into sugar in the bloodstream; also, avoid any vegetables that come packaged with premade sauce containing sugar, fat, or excess salt. In addition, deep-fried veggies, such as onion rings, tempura vegetables, and fried zucchini, should be reserved for special occasions only and eaten in small quantities.

Fruits

Like vegetables, fruits are high in fiber and nutrients. Fruits contain natural, healthful sugars, and the fiber content slows the sugars' absorption. Almost all fruits are good choices: fresh apples, oranges, pears, mangos, and melons are just a few options.

If you are following the DASH diet for weight loss, there are a few fruits to limit, with avocados leading the way, as they are high in fat and calories. In addition, limit consumption of dried fruits with added sugar by measuring portions ahead of time rather than eating straight from the package.

When choosing canned fruit, opt for fruits packed in water or their own juice rather than in syrup, which contains loads of added sugar. For example, pineapple packed in heavy syrup rather than water comes in at more than double the calorie count per serving. A one-cup portion packed in water contains 79 calories, while the equivalent servings packed in light and heavy syrup contain 131 and 198 calories, respectively.

Low-Fat Dairy Products

Not only are low-fat or fat-free dairy products high in calcium and protein, they contain a number of key nutrients, including vitamins A, D, and E as well as B_1, B_2, B_6, and B_{12}. In addition, low-fat and nonfat dairy products are very satisfying.

While you can enjoy a wide range of dairy products, there are some you'll want to limit or avoid entirely, even though they may be low-fat or fat-free. This includes yogurts with added sugar, and cheese products that are made with high amounts of salt or other additives. Desserts like ice cream and frozen yogurt are nice as an occasional treat; however, consuming these products regularly can undermine your DASH diet goals.

Nuts, Seeds, and Legumes

While many healthful eating plans place nuts, seeds, and legumes in other categories, they play such a vital role in the DASH diet for weight loss that we've put them in a category by themselves. These foods contain highly concentrated amounts of protein and fiber, and though legumes contain only a trace of natural fat, nuts and seeds contain high levels of heart-healthful fats, which are ideal for your health.

As with other foods, it's important to be selective when choosing which nuts, seeds, and legumes to eat. Limit or avoid highly processed versions, such as roasted and salted sunflower seeds, heavily salted or smoked nuts, and any nuts or seeds with candy coatings. In addition, since these items are relatively high in calories, be sure to measure out exact portions rather than snacking straight from a bag, jar, or tin. Being mindful of serving size makes it more difficult to overeat, particularly if you have a tendency to snack while working, watching TV, or driving.

Legumes serve as a vital protein source for vegetarians, and because they are easily adapted to recipes, they are an excellent alternative to meat, fish, and eggs for those who want to reduce their consumption of animal protein. If you are not already eating legumes on a regular basis, it's best to begin slowly and gradually increase the number of servings you consume each week. Many people overdo it in the beginning, only to end up with uncomfortable, embarrassing gas problems. If you tend to suffer from excessive flatulence after consuming legumes, consider using an enzyme-based product, such as Beano.

Legumes such as lentils, chickpeas (garbanzo beans), split peas, and soybeans are low in fat, yet they are rich in complex carbohydrates, protein, fiber, and minerals. Pairing legumes with whole grains like brown rice provides your body with a complete protein, which is more nutritious than legumes eaten on their own. Some grains to try with legumes include bulgur, whole-grain pasta, barley, quinoa, and even corn.

Meat, Poultry, Fish, Eggs, and Vegetable Proteins

Many types of meat contain high levels of saturated fat and cholesterol; they are also high in calories and low in volume. While using the DASH diet for weight loss, and for maintaining a healthful weight after the extra pounds are gone, it is recommended that you drastically reduce the amount of meat you eat; however, nothing is completely off-limits.

HOW MUCH MEAT EQUALS ONE SERVING?

Type of Meat	Serving Size
Cooked fish or shellfish	3 ounces
Chicken or turkey breast, skinless	3 ounces
Eggs and egg whites	3 whole eggs or 6 egg whites
Lean beef or pork	3 ounces
Low-fat deli meat	3 ounces

The best choices in this category are lean cuts of beef or pork, skinless chicken or turkey breast, fish, whole eggs or egg whites, lean deli meats, and low-fat soy products. Shop carefully for these items, as many contain additives, such as salt or MSG; some, particularly processed deli meats, even contain added sugar.

If you choose vegetarian proteins, keep an eye out for added sugar, salt, and fat. Textured vegetable protein (TVP) and plain tofu are good choices since they are easy to use and they readily absorb flavors from spices, vinegars, and other seasonings.

Eggs do contain cholesterol, but not so much that you can't enjoy them. Whole eggs are quick and easy to prepare, and you can consume as many as five per week without adversely affecting your weight-loss progress. You can also enjoy as many egg whites as you like, either by separating the whites from the yolks prior to cooking them or by choosing an egg white product, such as Egg Beaters, which is excellent for making scrambled eggs, omelets, and baked goods.

Fats, Oils, and Other Additives

Salad dressings, marinades, and condiments can enliven food wonderfully. The problem is that many commercially produced food additives and toppings contain unhealthful fats, high levels of sugar, and loads of salt, not to mention preservatives and other chemicals that do nothing to promote weight loss or bring about optimal health.

Butter, olive oil, and other fats do have their place; however, it is vital that you limit these items while losing weight, particularly since they are highly caloric. It's also important to select the right kinds of fats. For example, extra-virgin olive oil is one of the most desirable fats you can consume since it improves HDL (good) cholesterol levels. It is excellent in homemade salad dressings and is adaptable enough for use in many recipes.

Of all fats, the very worst are trans fats, which are added to commercially produced foods of many kinds in order to provide homogenization and to lengthen shelf life. Health care professionals recommend completely eliminating them from your diet, as they are synthetic substances that have been directly linked to serious health problems, including elevated LDL (bad) cholesterol levels, clogged arteries, and interference with the body's metabolic processes.

Foods that typically contain trans fats include:

- Certain cereals

- Deep-fried meats and fish

- Donuts

- French fries

- Many commercially produced cookies and crackers

- Margarine

- Nondairy creamer

- Peanut butter other than "natural" peanut butter, which separates into layers in the jar

- Potato chips

Avoiding foods that contain trans fats is as simple as reading the label: if a product contains hydrogenated vegetable oil or partially hydrogenated vegetable oil, it also contains trans fats. To avoid consuming trans fats while dining out, steer clear of bakery items and fried foods.

One of the biggest keys to DASH-diet success is to focus on eating all the *right* foods, instead of worrying too much about what *not* to eat. Taking a positive approach to eating will help you remain motivated and enthusiastic about the changes you're making in your life.

Fat-free Greek yogurt has a smooth, creamy texture and a delightfully tangy flavor— plus it has twice the protein of regular fat-free yogurt. It is an excellent replacement for other, fattier dairy items commonly used in recipes or preferred as condiments. For example, it's a good stand-in for sour cream and an excellent substitute for mayonnaise. And when strained of its liquid to make yogurt cheese, it serves as a great replacement for cream cheese and even butter.

CHAPTER EIGHT

Ten Steps for Success

Prepare to Succeed

Changing the way you eat can sometimes prove difficult, particularly when food is everywhere, making the refusal of old, unhealthful favorites all the more challenging. If this is your first time following a structured eating plan—or if you've tried other diets, only to lose momentum and eventually give up, ultimately regaining the lost weight plus a few more pounds—you may be wondering if you'll be able to stick with the DASH diet.

Though you may have to work hard to acquire new eating behaviors, like portion control, eating slowly, and saying no to foods that don't offer the nutrition, they will eventually become habits. As you begin to notice positive changes taking place within your body, you will feel increasingly motivated to continue with the plan. So long as you keep eating the healthiest foods available, the benefits that come with following the DASH diet will continue. No matter what your circumstances, you'll find that the ten steps presented here are valuable tools to keep you moving forward with your new healthful lifestyle while bypassing dietary roadblocks with ease.

Step One: Lay a Foundation for Success

Begin by creating a positive environment for yourself. The food environment most Americans live in is toxic in many ways, so eliminating sources of temptation from the start can help you avoid pitfalls. Clear your cupboards and refrigerator of unhealthful choices. In addition, do as much prep work as possible ahead of time; try chopping vegetables before you need them, pack lunches and snacks in the evening, and divide large packages of food into portions for easy access. Most important, remind yourself that *you* are the one who is in control of the food that goes into your mouth. Your health is ultimately in your own hands.

Step Two: Keep Thoughts Positive

When faced with temptation, telling yourself that for the sake of your health you are electing not to consume those donuts, that birthday cake, or that jumbo serving of fries, is a smarter strategy than reinforcing "I can't have that." Consider creating a short list of the reasons you are following the DASH diet. Keep a copy in your wallet or purse, post a copy on your refrigerator, and keep another one at your desk. Refer to it whenever the urge to make an unhealthful choice arises.

Step Three: Address Emotional Eating Issues

There are all sorts of reasons we eat and drink to excess. Most of us have celebrated milestones, mourned losses, and coped with stress by consuming certain foods, and for many of us, overindulgence happens too frequently. Worst of all, the foods on which we tend to binge are fatty, salty, and sugary; yet the comfort they provide is temporary. If you have a tendency to eat mindlessly as a way of coping with stress or emotions, address the problem head on. There is no shame in seeking professional counseling if needed. In addition, journaling, talking to a friend, or even exercising are positive replacements for unhealthful emotional eating.

Step Four: Make Time to Exercise

Now that you know why exercise is such an important factor in health, weight loss, and eliminating hypertension, make time for it in your daily life. One of the easiest ways to build more movement into your day is to get up thirty minutes earlier, put your shoes on your feet, and go for a morning walk before starting the rest of your daily routine. You'll feel more energetic, your desire for caffeine may decrease, and you will feel fantastic all day knowing that you kept an important promise to yourself first thing in the morning.

Step Five: Keep a Food and Exercise Diary

Keeping a food and exercise diary is a quick and simple way to stay on track. All you need is a small notebook you can carry with you; there are also smartphone apps available for keeping track of daily intake and exercise. Each time you eat something, write it down. Note any exercise you did, and for how long. Be honest about what and how much you are eating and exercising. Periodically review this diary and reflect on why you made any less-than-ideal choices. Doing this regularly will help you to make better choices over time.

Step Six: Keep Healthful Choices Available

It's all too easy to just grab the first food you see. Keeping healthful choices within reach is an excellent way to help you make the right decisions with ease. Fill an attractive bowl with fruit and keep it on the countertop or kitchen table. Put snack-sized bags of baby carrots, celery sticks, sliced bell peppers, and other healthful quick bites in a conspicuous spot in your refrigerator. Keep good-for-you snacks on hand at all times so you're never without something nutritious to eat—that way, if a less desirable choice is offered, you'll find it that much easier to say, "No, thanks."

Step Seven: Plan Ahead for Dining Out and Special Occasions

Following the DASH diet doesn't mean you have to chain yourself to your kitchen or become a hermit. If you know you are going to be dining out or celebrating a special occasion, find out the available options ahead of time. Restaurants often publish their menus online, so it's easy for you to determine what to order before you even arrive. If you desire an old favorite or really want to indulge in a rich dessert, make room for that treat in your daily eating plan. Enjoy every bite, knowing that you will be savoring healthier options at your next meal. Consider sharing a special appetizer or dessert with others—after all, food is always best when shared!

Step Eight: Say No to Food Pushers

Some of the people in your life may habitually offer you unhealthful foods, and saying no can feel difficult, especially when you're just beginning to form new habits. Create a standard response to offers of food; for example, "No, thank you, I've made a commitment to eating healthier and I will have to pass." You can also minimize contact with diet saboteurs, opting to spend time with them only in situations where food will not be present. If all else fails, consider addressing the problem directly by making a statement like: "I need to recover my health. Please help me by keeping tempting food away."

Step Nine: Think Progress Instead of Perfection

Whether your goal is to lose weight, eliminate hypertension, or just enjoy better health, aspire to progress rather than worrying too much about perfection. Don't beat yourself up if your goal for the month was to lose six pounds and you only lost four or five; instead, celebrate the win and keep moving forward. As with all endeavors in life, there will be ups and downs along the way. As long as you're continually making better choices and moving steadily toward your ultimate goal, you are making progress, and that's what really counts.

Step Ten: Forgive Mistakes and Start Over

If you've binged on an entire half-gallon of ice cream, eaten donuts for breakfast for a whole week, or made other poor choices, forgive yourself for the error. Resolve to do better next time and just start over, reminding yourself of the many reasons the changes you are making are worthwhile. One of the saddest mistakes people make after botching a new eating plan is to give up completely, thinking that they are doomed to a life of unhealthful habits. Instead of following in their footsteps, think about why the mistake occurred and watch for similar pitfalls in the future.

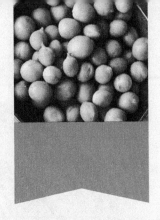

PART **FOUR**

DASH Diet in Action

Chapter Nine DASH Diet Eating Guide

Chapter Ten DASH-Friendly Cooking Methods

Chapter Eleven 30-Day Meal Plan for Health and Weight Loss

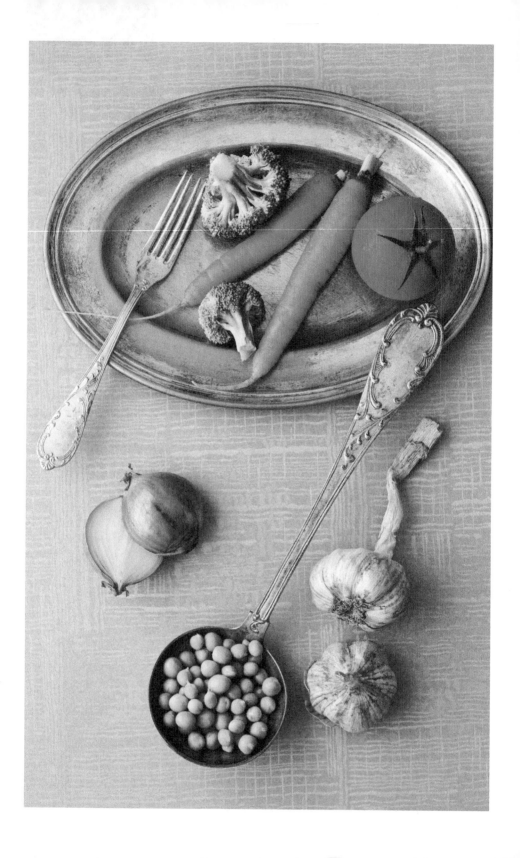

DASH Diet Eating Guide

DASH in Action

Now that you know which foods are the most nutritious and beneficial to your dietary goals, plan to use them in place of the unhealthful options that lurk on supermarket shelves, in vending machines, and in your own pantry. Beyond just knowing which foods are best for you, it's important that you take a look at your daily eating habits and resolve to eat your meals with intention.

Creating Healthful Eating Habits

What does your daily food intake look like now? For those consuming a typical American diet, breakfast often consists of coffee, juice, and a sugary muffin or donut, or perhaps a fast-food breakfast sandwich. Lunch is often eaten on the run—more fast food: perhaps a burger and fries or a burrito, washed down with a soda. Dinner is frequently quick and convenient, and more often than not, it's eaten in front of the television. Pizza, fried chicken, and takeout meals are American favorites. Snacks often consist of vending-machine fare: candy, highly processed baked goods, and salt-laden chips or pretzels. These high-calorie treats might be consumed throughout the day, although many people also snack after dinner while watching TV.

No matter what your diet looks like now, you can change it for the better simply by replacing unhealthful habits with good ones.

- Breakfast—For breakfast, enjoy a coffee if you like, but reduce the size and modify what you put in it. Use low-fat or nonfat milk instead of half-and-half, and limit the sugar. Stay away from prepared coffee drinks—order it black instead so you control what is added. Have a nourishing breakfast that you enjoy—oatmeal, eggs, and cereal with milk are some excellent choices.

- Midmorning snack—Even if you're not a big snacker, consider planning healthful snacks throughout the day. Good choices include almonds, cheese, vegetables, and fruits. These will help you stay satisfied and prevent overeating later in the day.

- Lunch—For lunch, enjoy salads or sandwiches made with healthful items such as low-sodium deli meat, low-fat cheese, and plenty of lettuce, tomatoes, and other vegetables. Be sure to choose whole-grain bread for your sandwiches. Low-sodium soups and stews are also great choices, as are leftovers from the healthful meal you enjoyed the night before.

- Midafternoon snack—Enjoy another healthful snack midway between lunch-time and dinner. You'll enjoy improved energy throughout the afternoon, and you won't be famished when it's finally time to sit down at the dinner table.

- Dinner—Don't be afraid to have fun with your final meal of the day. Select a protein such as chicken breast, fish, and the occasional lean cut of beef or pork. Pair it with your favorite vegetables and whole-grain pasta or bread. For complex flavor that doesn't add calories, season dishes with fresh herbs and a variety of spices. Enjoy fruit for dessert on most days, reserving ice cream, cake, and other sugary items for special occasions.

- Evening snack—If you feel the need to have a snack after dinner, be sure it's a healthful one. Air-popped popcorn, vegetables and hummus, or fruit are good options. A hot cup of herbal tea before bedtime is also a satisfying option.

- Fluid intake—Ensure that you are drinking enough healthful liquids through-out each day—particularly water. Thirst often masquerades as hunger, and providing your body with the water it requires can help to prevent overeat-ing. In addition, staying properly hydrated supports a healthful metabolism. Drinking eight 8-ounce glasses of water is usually sufficient. If you are exercis-ing more, or if the weather is hot, you may need more fluid each day.

The healthier the eating habits you embrace, the more benefits you will realize. Most unhealthful habits are formed over a long period of time—for example, maybe you stopped by a fast-food place for lunch one day when you were in a hurry, and you soon found yourself stopping there repeatedly. Before you knew it, that fast-food lunch was a habit—one, perhaps, you were hardly aware of.

Establishing smart eating habits is an intentional process that requires some willpower at first. Engage yourself in the process of shopping for new foods, prepar-ing your own meals and snacks, and truly enjoying each meal. Eat slowly and savor the entire experience, reminding yourself of the benefits you'll receive by consuming foods that are good for your body. Soon, you will find that old, negative patterns have been replaced by new, positive ones.

To change any habit, you must first be aware that it exists—be honest with yourself. Keeping a food diary will help you to spot detrimental eating habits and to pinpoint trends, such as workday versus weekend practices. Once you know which habits you'd like to change, take small steps that are easy to repeat and execute those steps with intention. Everyone is different, but establishing a new habit usually takes twenty-one to thirty days. Each time you make a good food choice, you are reinforcing the habits you wish to maintain, while simultaneously eliminating the negative habits you'd like to replace.

Focus on Feelings: The Mind-Body Connection and Intentional Eating

In the past, you may have overlooked feelings that have arisen before, during, and after meals and snacks. Perhaps you ate or drank to numb feelings that were uncomfortable for you. Focusing on feelings and really paying attention to what your body is telling you will help you to eat intentionally. In turn, you will enjoy even greater success with the DASH diet.

Begin by deciding to notice when you feel hungry or thirsty. Next, think about which healthful food or beverage you should consume to satiate your appetite. If you are feeling stressed out or emotional, consider whether it is necessary to eat the food you are craving or reach for an alcoholic beverage to soothe yourself—also consider how you'll feel after you've had it. Will you regret the decision and be disappointed in yourself? Keep in mind that clever marketing experts use the mind-body connection to convince you that food will fulfill emotional needs when, in fact, the exact opposite is true.

Finally, remind yourself why you've decided to change your eating habits in the first place. Appreciate the foods you eat, not just for their flavor, but also for the nutrients that fuel your body. Imagine the way you will look and feel once you have achieved your goals—and after you've eaten the meal or snack you planned for yourself, notice the feeling of satisfaction and pride that follows.

Paying attention to what your body is telling you will help you identify the difference between true physical hunger and unaddressed emotional needs. When you are tempted to diverge from your eating plan, remind yourself that a warm cup of herbal tea, a conversation with a friend, a short walk, or some cuddle time with a pet will go much further than will food or alcohol in helping to alleviate feelings of stress, sadness, boredom, anxiety, or other troubling emotions. The numbing properties that comfort food and drink provide are only temporary. On the other hand, meaningful, intentional actions that deal directly with what's going on internally can truly alleviate emotional hunger.

When combined, fat and sugar encourage emotional eating and can lead to binges. To conquer serious cravings, particularly when you are feeling stressed or anxious, choose a healthful snack high in antioxidants. Fresh strawberries contain only 8 calories per ounce. They nourish and hydrate the body, and are a perfect substitute for options that will likely result in sluggishness. Purple grapes, blueberries, bananas, and other fruits are also excellent choices.

Empowering yourself with knowledge about food and fitting it into its proper place in your life will propel you toward success. Review recipes each week, create a daily menu, and shop accordingly. You'll find that taking a methodical approach to eating simplifies your routine and makes avoiding pitfalls much simpler.

CHAPTER TEN

DASH-Friendly Cooking Methods

The DASH Diet Cook

Following the DASH diet does not have to be boring, and cooking the foods you'll be eating on this plan is easy, especially when you have the right tools on hand.

Selecting the Right Cookware

There are a few simple pans and appliances that make cooking for the DASH diet all the more manageable. You may already have these items in your kitchen; if not, you'll find they are inexpensive and easy to find in stores.

- Nonstick cookware—Instead of traditional cast-iron or stainless steel cookware, select nonstick pots and pans that free you from having to add extra fat to your food to prevent it from sticking.

- Rice cooker—A rice cooker is great for cooking large amounts of rice and other whole grains; it cooks food to perfection and allows you to make large batches with minimal effort.

- Vegetable steamer—A basket-shaped vegetable steamer insert makes preparing vegetables easy, plus steaming vegetables rather than boiling them helps them retain nutrients.

Some other items that make cooking a breeze include nonstick baking pans, blenders, and food processors.

Using Spices Instead of Salt

There are many fantastic low-salt or no-salt spice blends on the market; in addition, fresh herbs such as basil, dill, and cilantro add zip to foods without adding fat, salt, or calories. You can also use vinegar, onions, garlic, ginger, or fruit to add flavor to dishes.

Broiling

Broiling is a fast, easy cooking method that works well with lean cuts of meat, fish, and poultry, and it can be used to finish vegetables as well. You will need a broiler pan or a wire rack placed on a rimmed baking sheet. Lining the lower portion of the broiler pan with foil to catch drips will help save on cleanup time, and using marinades or rubs will add wonderful flavor to the foods you prepare in this way.

Steaming

Steaming food requires no additional fat. While it is most commonly used for preparing vegetables, you can steam fish, chicken, and meat as well. When steaming foods, it is important to ensure the pot never goes dry. You can toss a few clean coins or marbles into the bottom of the pan before adding the steamer insert. These will make noise as the liquid boils; if the water level drops, the noise will stop, reminding you to add more water.

Adding olive oil to vegetables or other foods just after steaming will add immense flavor, along with a smidge of healthful fat. Even ½ teaspoon of olive oil will provide more satisfying flavor than would sautéing the food in a tablespoon of fat. Top with fresh, chopped herbs for an even more sensational flavor boost.

Poaching

Poaching is another simple, no-fat-added technique that works well for cooking a wide variety of foods. Eggs, chicken, and fish are all excellent candidates for poaching, either in water, a bit of wine, or some low-sodium broth. You will need a large, flat-bottomed pan with a tight-fitting lid; place the food in the pan, adding just enough liquid to cover it. Bring it to a gentle simmer so that barely any bubbles break the surface. Watch closely and don't allow the liquid to boil, since this can cause foods to become tough. Save the cooking liquid if you like; it makes a nice base for soups.

Wrapping

Wrapping food in parchment paper before baking allows it to steam gently in its own juices, preventing dryness and flavor loss. This method is excellent for chicken and fish, and is ideal for minimizing cleanup. Simply place the food on a large piece of parchment paper, along with any spices or vegetables you wish to add. Wrap it up loosely, folding open edges to create a sealed pouch. Place the package on a rimmed baking sheet and set on the oven rack. Be sure to use only oven-safe parchment paper; do not substitute waxed paper.

Pureeing

Pureeing cooked vegetables transforms them into a velvety, delicious treat. Sweet potatoes, cauliflower, and squash are perfect candidates for this treatment. First simmer or steam the vegetables until tender, then blend them with a small amount of broth until you achieve the desired consistency. Because hot liquids expand, fill the blender only halfway, using a potholder or towel to keep the lid firmly in place while the machine is running. If you love the idea of creating thick, creamy soups, consider purchasing an immersion blender, which can be submerged in a pot of hot liquid for quick, easy pureeing.

Baking

Baking foods at high heat helps to deepen natural flavors. A baked medley of root vegetables is a comforting side dish for a cold evening; parsnips, carrots, sweet onions, and even brussels sprouts take on delicious complexity and sweetness when baked. Baking works well for chicken, fish, and meat, too; be sure to baste foods with liquid during baking to prevent them from drying out.

Grilling or Barbecuing

Grilling is an uncomplicated way to prepare flavorful dishes of all kinds. Fish, shrimp, meat, and poultry are all fantastic for the grill, as are vegetables. If you like the idea of preparing your food alfresco, invest in some special tools to make low-fat grilling simple and mess-free. A fish basket, a vegetable tray, and some kebab skewers are just some of the inexpensive, easy-to-find tools that can take your grilling to the next level while keeping unwanted fat out of your food.

CHAPTER ELEVEN

30-Day Meal Plan for Health and Weight Loss

Jump into DASH

It is often difficult to start a new diet or make a lifestyle choice because eating habits are very hard to break and many diets seem to have more restrictions than choices. As with any other diet it is important to use the freshest ingredients possible when preparing your meals. If you need to purchase any processed ingredients such as frozen or canned produce, always study the nutrition labels carefully to ensure that you know exactly what is in the food. Pay particular attention to the sodium, fat, additives, and sugar content to make sure these amounts are within the DASH parameters. Also watch serving sizes because even when the food is healthful for you, overeating is overeating!

Following an easy 30-day meal plan to start is great way to get on the right track and become familiar with the DASH diet guidelines. The 30-day DASH meal plan is calculated on a 2,000 calorie per day diet, allowing 1,500 mg of sodium daily, and designed for one person. Keep in mind that the DASH diet will be a lifestyle choice not just a quick fix to fit into a favorite dress or pair of pants for an upcoming special event. You will find that most of the foods on the plan are familiar and easy to find in your local grocery store. Pick recipes that suit your taste, culinary skill level and routine so that the DASH diet fits successfully into your life.

If you need to adjust the calories up or down, remember to follow these tips:

- If you need to lower your calories, decrease your servings of grains and fruits by one or two each.

- If you need to raise your calorie intake, increase your fruits and vegetables first, then grains.

Note: Dishes marked with a star (*) are provided in the recipe section.

Day 1

BREAKFAST

Oatmeal with Pistachios and Currants*

LUNCH

Basil Chicken Wrap
- 1 medium tortilla
- 3 ounces cooked, chopped chicken breast
- ½ cup halved green grapes
- 1 tablespoon pecan pieces
- 1 tablespoon plain fat-free yogurt

1 tomato, sliced

1 cup fat-free milk

SNACK

1½ cups broccoli or cauliflower florets with a splash of balsamic vinegar

DINNER

Coconut Fish Stew*

Day 2

BREAKFAST

1 light multigrain English muffin
- 1 tablespoon almond butter
- ½ cup sliced strawberries

1 cup vanilla fat-free yogurt
- 1 tablespoon unsalted sunflower seeds

1 cup apple juice

LUNCH

Crunchy Chicken Salad*

SNACK

Thai Pork in Lettuce Wraps*

DINNER

Baked Salmon with Mango Salsa
- 4 ounces salmon fillet sautéed in
- ½ teaspoon olive oil and cook at 450 degrees F for 15–20 minutes.
- Mango Salsa (¼ ripe mango diced, ¼ red pepper diced, ¼ cup diced cucumber, ½ scallion, sliced)

½ cup wild rice
1 cup lightly blanched fresh asparagus

Day 3

BREAKFAST

Hollywood Broiled Grapefruit*

LUNCH

Waldorf Tuna Salad
- 3 ounces drained, unsalted water-packed tuna
- 2 tablespoons plain fat-free yogurt
- ½ cup halved green grapes
- 2 stalks celery, diced
- 2 cups baby spinach
- 1 tablespoon low-sodium low-fat feta cheese
- Squeeze of fresh lemon juice

Herbal iced tea or sparkling water

SNACK

Turkey Quesadillas*

DINNER

Grilled Halibut with Roasted Red Pepper Salsa
- 6 ounce halibut filet, grilled until cooked through, turning once, about 8 minutes per side brushed with 1 teaspoon olive oil
- ½ cup chopped roasted red pepper
- ½ cup halved cherry tomatoes
- 1 green onion, chopped
- 1 tablespoon chopped fresh basil
- ½ teaspoon fresh lime juice
- ¼ teaspoon minced garlic

1 cup lightly blanched asparagus
1 cup cooked basmati rice
1 cup skim milk

Day 4

BREAKFAST

1 small whole-wheat pita with
- 2 tablespoons sodium-free peanut butter
1 medium peach
1 cup fat-free milk
Decaffeinated coffee or herbal tea

LUNCH

Homemade Tomato Soup*

SNACK

1 cup fat-free yogurt
2 plums
1 tablespoon raw sunflower seeds

DINNER

Portobello Stroganoff over Egg Noodles*

Day 5

BREAKFAST

Egg White Omelet*

LUNCH

Pasta Salad
- 1 cup cooked whole-wheat or rice pasta
- 1 small tomato, chopped
- ½ cup sliced mushrooms
- ½ yellow pepper, seeded and chopped
- ⅓ cup chopped red onion
- 2 tablespoons low-fat, low-sodium feta cheese
1 cup fresh fruit juice

⅓ cup low-fat cottage cheese
½ cup blueberries
1 tablespoon pumpkin seeds

DINNER

Best Practices Roast Chicken*

Day 6

BREAKFAST

Strawberry Waffles
- 2 whole-grain waffles
- ¼ cup fat-free cottage cheese
- 1 cup sliced strawberries
- 2 tablespoons slivered almonds

1 cup herbal tea or decaffeinated coffee

LUNCH

Waldorf Chicken Salad
- 3 ounces cooked chopped chicken
- 3 stalks celery, diced
- 1 small tart apple, cored and chopped
- ½ cup halved green grapes
- 3 tablespoons fat-free plain yogurt
- 1 tablespoon dried cranberries

1 cup cantaloupe cubes
1 cup herbal iced tea

SNACK

Agua Fresca*

DINNER

Turkey Chili with Black Beans*

Day 7

BREAKFAST

Cucumber and Ricotta Open-Faced Sandwiches*

LUNCH

Crab Papaya Salad
- 3 ounces real crab meat
- 2 cups baby spinach leaves
- 1 large papaya, peeled, seeded and sliced into strips
- 1 cup cherry tomatoes
- ½ yellow pepper, seeded and chopped finely
- ½ cup cucumber slices
- 3 thin slices of red onion
- 2 tablespoons chopped cilantro
- 2 tablespoons red wine vinaigrette

Herbal iced tea

SNACK

Baked Applesauce with Walnuts*

DINNER

Barbecued Beef Kebabs
- 3 ounces of beef, cubed and threaded onto wood skewers with
- 1 cup mixed vegetable chunks (red pepper, mushrooms, onion, and zucchini) and barbecued until cooked the desired doneness, about 6 minutes per side for medium

½ cup cooked brown rice
½ cup peas (fresh or frozen)
1 large orange
1 cup cranberry juice

Day 8

BREAKFAST

¾ cup cooked quinoa (cooked with ½ cup skim milk and 1 cup water)
- ½ cup unsweetened applesauce
- 2 tablespoons pecans

½ whole-wheat pita with
- 1 teaspoon almond or nut butter

1 banana

Herbal tea

LUNCH

Portobello Mushroom Burgers
- 1 large Portobello mushroom (grilled on the barbeque until soft)
- 1 whole-wheat burger bun
- 1 tablespoon goat cheese
- ½ small tomato sliced
- 1 slice red onion
- 2 Bibb lettuce leaves

1 cup baby carrots
- ¼ cup fat-free ranch dressing

1 cup skim milk

SNACK

Cajun Popcorn*

DINNER

Shrimp with Jalapeño-Orange Sauce over Pasta*

Day 9

BREAKFAST

DASH Migas*

LUNCH

Vegetable and Hummus Pita*

SNACK

2 celery stalks smeared with
2 teaspoons salt-free peanut butter
¼ cup raisins

DINNER

"Spaghetti" with Fresh Tomato Sauce
- 2 cups carrot noodles (strips of carrot made with a peeler) tossed with
- 2 large tomatoes, chopped
- ½ cup artichoke hearts, quartered
- 1 teaspoon chopped fresh basil
- 1 tablespoon grated Parmesan cheese
- Pinch red chili pepper flakes

2 cups chopped romaine
- 1 tablespoon low-fat Caesar dressing

1 cup melon, cubed

Sparkling water or herbal iced tea

Day 10

BREAKFAST

Mango Blast Smoothie*

LUNCH

Grilled Chicken Breast on Mixed Green Salad
- 1 grilled 4 ounce chicken breast, sliced
- 3 cups of fresh mixed baby greens
- ¼ small red onion, peeled and sliced thinly
- ½ cup sliced strawberries
- ⅓ cup slivered almonds
- 3 teaspoons reduced-fat balsamic vinaigrette

1 whole-wheat flatbread

1 cup fat-free milk

SNACK

10 whole-grain low-sodium crackers

½ cup hummus

DINNER

Panko-Crusted Chicken Fingers with Apricot Dipping Sauce*

Day 11

BREAKFAST

1 slice toasted whole-wheat bread
1 hard-boiled egg, sliced
1 small tomato, sliced
½ ounce low-fat cheese, shredded
½ grapefruit
1 cup skim milk

LUNCH

Chicken Curry*

SNACK

Strawberry-Mango Salsa with Basil*

DINNER

Baked Maple Salmon with Braised Spinach
- 4 ounce salmon fillet drizzled with
- 1 teaspoon pure maple syrup topped with
- 1 teaspoon sesame seeds and baked at 450 degrees F for 10 minutes
- 2 bunches spinach, washed and tossed in 1 tablespoon water in a large skillet over medium heat until wilted and bright green
- ½ green onion, thinly sliced on a bias
1 cup fresh squeezed lemonade

Day 12

BREAKFAST

1 cup fresh mixed fruits of your choice, mixed with
- 1 cup fat-free, low-calorie yogurt
- ½ cup slivered almonds
1 piece whole-grain toast
1 teaspoon almond or nut butter
1 cup fat-free milk
Black decaffeinated coffee or herbal tea

LUNCH

Chicken Stuffed Red Pepper
- 1 large red pepper (top cut off, seeded, and baked until soft in at 350 degrees F, about 5 minutes)
- ½ cup brown rice, cooked
- 4 ounces shredded chicken breast
- 1 small tomato, seeded and diced
- 1 green onion, chopped
- ¼ teaspoon minced garlic
- ½ teaspoon chopped fresh basil
- 2 tablespoons low-fat cheese, shredded

2 kiwis

1 cup skim milk

SNACK

Shrimp and Mango "Ceviche"*

DINNER

Pan-Seared Whitefish on Lemony Quinoa*

Day 13

BREAKFAST

Pumpkin or Sweet Potato Oatmeal*

LUNCH

Vegetable and Mozzarella Frittata*

SNACK

1 apple
1 ounce low-fat cheese

DINNER

Oven Roasted Chicken Breast
- 4 ounce chicken breast, baked at 350 degrees F for 20 minutes
- Cracked black pepper

Baked sweet potato
- 1 teaspoon unsalted butter
- Sprinkle of cinnamon

Arugula Salad
- 1 cup baby arugula
- ½ cup halved cherry tomatoes
- ½ cup sliced cucumber
- 1 tablespoon balsamic vinegar

1 cup skim milk

Day 14

BREAKFAST

1 cup fresh-squeezed orange juice
1 whole-wheat bagel
- 2 tablespoons light cream cheese
- 1 small tomato sliced

1 cup cubed melon

LUNCH

Simple Rosemary Salmon*

SNACK

1 slice whole-grain toast
1 tablespoon almond butter
½ small banana, sliced

DINNER

Quick Vegetarian Ramen Noodle Soup*

Day 15

BREAKFAST

Substantial Fruit Salad*

LUNCH

Turkey Burgers with Cranberry-Scallion Sauce*

SNACK

3 cups air-popped unsalted popcorn

DINNER

Pork Fajitas
- ¼ pound pork tenderloin, cut into strips tossed with
- Spice mix (½ teaspoon chili powder, ⅛ teaspoon paprika, pinch of ground coriander, pinch of garlic powder)
- ½ small onion, sliced thinly
- ½ red pepper, seeded and sliced thinly
- ½ yellow pepper, seeded and sliced thinly
- 2 whole-wheat flour tortillas, warmed in the microwave
- 1 medium tomato, diced
- 1 cup shredded lettuce
- ¼ cup shredded low-fat cheddar cheese

1 large mango, peeled, pitted, and cut into chunks

1 cup sparkling water

Day 16

BREAKFAST

French Toast
- 2 slices whole-wheat bread
- 1 egg
- 1 teaspoon unsalted butter
- Dash of cinnamon
- 1 cup fresh raspberries
- 2 tablespoons plain fat-free yogurt

1 cup herbal tea or decaffeinated coffee

LUNCH

Mango Jicama Salad
- ½ cup cooked shredded pork
- ½ cup torn lettuce leaves
- ½ large mango, peeled, pitted, and sliced into thin strips
- ½ large red pepper, seeded and cut into thin strips
- ½ small jicama, peeled and grated coarsely
- 1 small carrot, peeled and grated

- ½ cup bean sprouts
- 2 tablespoons toasted sesame seeds
- 1 tablespoon chopped coriander

1 cup unsweetened pineapple juice

SNACK

Roasted Red Pepper Dip*

DINNER

Vegetable Lasagna*

Day 17

BREAKFAST

Fruit Kebabs
- 1 cup assorted fruit chunks (strawberries, melon, banana, pear, apple or pineapple)
- 2 ounces low-fat cheese, cut into chunks

1 whole-grain English muffin
- 2 tablespoons almond butter

1 cup herbal tea

LUNCH

Cold Soba Noodles with Peanut Sauce*

SNACK

1 small bunch of green grapes
1 ounce low-fat cheese

DINNER

Creamy Beans and Greens*

Day 18

BREAKFAST

Easy Breakfast Casserole with Vegetables*

LUNCH

Watermelon, Feta, and Mint Summer Salad*

SNACK

1 red pepper, seeded and cut into strips
¼ cup low-fat ranch dressing

DINNER

Pecan-Crusted Baked Halibut
- 4 ounces halibut
- 1 tablespoon crushed pecans

½ cup quinoa with
- ½ cup chopped tomato

½ cup fresh green beans, lightly blanched
1 cup fresh blueberries with chopped mint
Herbal iced tea or ice water

Day 19

BREAKFAST

Fruit Parfaits
- 1 cup mixed fresh fruit
- ½ cup fat-free vanilla yogurt
- ¼ cup low-fat granola

1 cup skim milk

LUNCH

Pasta Caprese*

SNACK

Vegetable Smoothie*

DINNER

Chicken Stir-Fry
- 3 ounces chicken breast, in strips
- 1 teaspoon sesame oil
- 1 teaspoon minced garlic

- ½ teaspoon grated fresh ginger
- 1 cup broccoli florets
- 1 small carrot, peeled and sliced thinly
- 1 cup snow peas
- ½ red pepper, cut into strips
- 1 green onion, sliced thinly

½ cup brown rice

1 cup sparkling water

- Squeeze of fresh lemon juice

Day 20

BREAKFAST

Fruit-Filled French Toast*

LUNCH

Salmon Salad
- 4 ounces cooked salmon
- 3 cups baby spinach
- 1 grapefruit, peeled and cut into segments
- 1 small ripe avocado, peeled, pitted, and sliced
- ½ cup halved cherry tomatoes
- 2 tablespoons oil and vinegar dressing
- 3 tablespoons chopped pistachios

1 slice pumpernickel bread

1 cup skim milk

SNACK

1 cup light strawberry yogurt, fat-free and sugar free

¼ cup cashews

DINNER

Grilled Pork Tenderloin with Garlic and Herbs*

Day 21

BREAKFAST

Egg White Breakfast Sandwich
- 1 whole-wheat bagel
- 2 scrambled egg whites
- 1 small tomato, sliced
- ½ cup baby spinach leaves
- 2 tablespoons shredded low-fat cheese

1 peach

1 cup herbal tea

LUNCH

Lightning Fast Chicken Stir-Fry*

SNACK

Red, White, and Blue Fruit Kebabs*

DINNER

Barbequed Honey Chili Shrimp Skewers
- 4 large shrimp, peeled and deveined
- ½ teaspoon olive oil
- Juice and zest 1 lime
- Black pepper to taste
- 1 teaspoon honey
- Pinch of ground chili powder
- Pinch of paprika

1 baked sweet potato
- Pinch of ground cinnamon

1 cup lightly blanched peas

Day 22

BREAKFAST

Spanish-Style Scrambled Eggs*

Curried Chicken Salad Pita Wrap
- 1 pita shell, cut in half
- 1 poached chicken breast (4 ounces), cut into cubes
- ½ cup fat-free yogurt
- ½ teaspoon curry powder
- 1 tablespoon fresh lime juice
- 1 stalk celery, chopped
- ½ tart apples, cored and diced
- 2 tablespoons dried cranberries

1 ripe mango, peeled, pitted, and sliced

1 cup skim milk

SNACK

1 ounce light cheese

1 cup baby carrots

DINNER

Argentinean-Style Flank Steak*

Day 23

BREAKFAST

Brown Rice Porridge
- 1 cup cooked brown rice
- ½ cup skim milk
- Drizzle of maple syrup
- Dash of cinnamon

1 cup berries

LUNCH

White Bean and Sage Soup*

SNACK

Cucumber and Dill Tea Sandwiches*

DINNER

Chicken Soft Taco
- 1 multigrain tortilla
- 4 ounces cooked chopped chicken
- ½ cup black beans
- ½ ripe avocado, sliced
- ½ small tomato, chopped
- ½ cup shredded iceberg lettuce

1 cup unsweetened applesauce

.1 cup herbal tea

Day 24

BREAKFAST

Breakfast Hash*

LUNCH

Moroccan Lentil Salad
- 1½ cup cooked lentils
- ½ cup chickpeas, rinsed and drained
- ½ small red pepper, seeded and chopped
- ½ small yellow pepper, seeded and chopped
- ½ cup halved cherry tomatoes
- ½ cup chopped cucumber
- 1 green onion, chopped
- ½ jalapeño pepper, minced
- Juice of 1 lime
- ¼ teaspoon ground cumin

Herbal iced tea

SNACK

Spice-Roasted Sunflower and Pumpkin Seeds*

DINNER

Grilled Pork Tenderloin
- 4 ounces grilled pork tenderloin rubbed with nutmeg and cinnamon

1 small baked potato
- 1 tablespoon fat-free plain yogurt
- 1 tablespoon sliced green onions

Mixed green salad
- 2 cups green-leaf lettuce
- ½ cup halved cherry tomatoes
- ½ cup cucumber slices
- ½ cup shredded carrot
- ½ red pepper, sliced
- 2 tablespoons balsamic vinaigrette

Day 25

BREAKFAST

Creamy "French" Scrambled Eggs*

LUNCH

Massaged Kale Salad*

SNACK

1 cup vanilla fat-free, low-calorie yogurt
4 graham crackers

DINNER

Baked Chicken with Moroccan Peach Salsa
- 1 chicken breast, browned in a pan over medium heat and baked at 350 degrees F until cooked through, about 25 minutes
- 1 ripe peach, pitted and chopped into large chunks
- ½ small red pepper, seeded and diced
- 1 scallion, chopped
- 2 tablespoons golden raisins
- ⅛ teaspoon ground cinnamon
- ⅛ teaspoon ground ginger
- Pinch of allspice

1 cup cooked quinoa
1 cup lightly blanched green beans

Day 26

BREAKFAST

Peanut Butter Smoothie
- 1 banana
- 2 tablespoons salt-free peanut butter
- ½ cup skim milk
- ½ cup fat-free vanilla yogurt

1 cup sliced strawberries

LUNCH

Roasted Vegetables on Ciabatta*

SNACK

Vegetable Chips*

DINNER

Cajun Spiced Salmon with Corn Salsa
- 6 ounces salmon fillet, rubbed with Cajun spice mix (½ teaspoon paprika, ⅛ teaspoon ground cumin, ⅛ teaspoon garlic powder and pinch cayenne) seared in a hot pan and baked at 450 degrees F for 10–15 minutes
- 1 cup salt-free corn kernels
- ¼ ripe avocado, chopped
- ½ small red pepper, seeded and chopped
- ½ scallion, chopped
- 1 teaspoon lime juice
- 1 teaspoon coarsely chopped fresh coriander

5 baby potatoes, blanched tender
- ¼ teaspoon sweet butter
- ½ teaspoon chopped dill

1 large tomato, sliced
- Splash of balsamic vinegar

Day 27

BREAKFAST

Yogurt and Tropical Fruit Parfaits*

Shaved Roast Beef Sandwich
- 1 whole-wheat bun
- ¼ pound shaved beef
- 1 ounce sliced low-fat cheese
- 2 thin red onion slices
- ¼ cup cucumber slices
- 1 teaspoon spicy mustard

1 large tart apple

1 cup skim milk

SNACK

Trail mix
- ¼ cup raisins or dried cranberries
- 2 tablespoons sunflower seeds
- ¼ cup roasted unsalted almonds

DINNER

Chicken Breasts with Mango-Rosemary Sauce on Brown Rice*

Day 28

BREAKFAST

1 cup bran flakes cereal
- 1 banana, sliced
- 1 cup skim milk

½ cup sliced strawberries
- 1 tablespoon plain fat-free yogurt
- 1 tablespoon sunflower seeds

1 cup fresh-squeezed orange juice

LUNCH

Greek Steak Pita Sandwiches
- ¼ flank steak, trimmed, seasoned with garlic, barbequed to medium, and tossed with lemon zest and juice from ½ small lemon and ½ teaspoon oregano
- 2 whole-wheat pitas
- 1 cup shredded romaine lettuce

- 1 small tomato, chopped
- ⅓ small red onion, peeled and sliced thinly
- 2 tablespoons low-fat, low-sodium feta cheese

2 cups cubed watermelon

1 cup skim milk

SNACK

Homemade Hummus with Crudités*

DINNER

Spicy Tofu Stir-Fry*

Day 29

BREAKFAST

Banana Oatmeal
- 1 cup traditionally cooked large-flake oatmeal
- 1 banana, sliced
- 2 tablespoons pecans
- 1 cup fat-free milk

1 cup mixed berries

LUNCH

Flattened Chicken on Arugula Salad*

SNACK

Baked Chili-Lime Tortilla Chips*

DINNER

Hearty Beef Chili simmered until heated through
- ¼ pound extra-lean ground beef
- ¼ cup chopped onion
- 1 large tomatoes, chopped
- ½ cup sodium-free kidney beans, rinsed and drained
- ½ cup sodium-free navy beans, rinsed and drained
- 1 stalk celery
- ½ green pepper, seeded and chopped

- ¼ jalapeño pepper, minced
- 1 tablespoon chili powder or to taste
  Topped with
- 1 tablespoon fat-free sour cream

1 cup unsweetened applesauce

1 cup herbal iced tea

Day 30

BREAKFAST

Breakfast Burrito*

LUNCH

Shrimp and Mango Wraps
- 3 large cooked shrimp, chopped
- 1 tablespoon fat-free sour cream
- ½ teaspoon minced jalapeño pepper
- ½ ripe mango, sliced
- ½ cup shredded lettuce

1 cup cubed melon

Sparkling water with a squeeze of fresh lemon

SNACK

1 large peach

½ cup roasted unsalted almonds

DINNER

Pot Roast with Sweet Potatoes, Peas, and Onions*

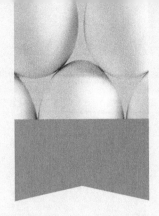

PART FIVE

150 DASH Recipes

Chapter Twelve DASH Breakfasts

Chapter Thirteen DASH Lunches

Chapter Fourteen DASH Snacks and Appetizers

Chapter Fifteen DASH Dinners

Chapter Sixteen DASH Desserts

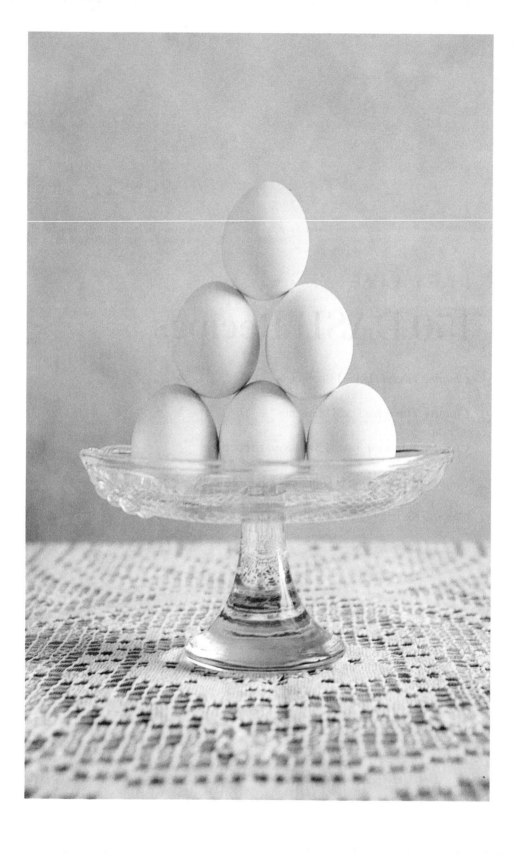

DASH Breakfasts

- ▶ Mango Blast Smoothie

- ▶ Green Tea and Banana Smoothie

- ▶ The Stomach Soother Smoothie

- ▶ The Green Monster

- ▶ Peach Berry Fizz

- ▶ Hollywood Broiled Grapefruit

- ▶ Yogurt and Tropical Fruit Parfaits

- ▶ Substantial Fruit Salad

- ▶ Oatmeal with Pistachios and Currants

- ▶ Sweet Potato Oatmeal

- ▶ Granola, Your Way

- ▶ Acorn Squash, Apple, and Peach "Pie"

- ▶ Folded French Omelet

- ▶ Egg White Omelet

- ▶ Creamy "French" Scrambled Eggs

- ▶ Spanish-Style Scrambled Eggs

- ▶ Baked Eggs with Truffle Oil and Fontina Cheese

- ▶ Perfect Poached Eggs with Lemon Sauce

- ▶ Easy Breakfast Casserole with Vegetables

- ▶ Crustless Spinach Quiche

- ▶ DASH Migas

- ▶ Grits and Eggs

- ▶ Egg Tart with Sweet Potato Crust

- ▶ Strawberry and Cream Cheese Cakes

- ▶ Cucumber and Ricotta Open-Face Sandwiches

- ▶ Hummus and Sardines on Toast

- ▶ Breakfast Burrito

- ▶ Fruit-Filled French Toast

- ▶ Breakfast Hash

- ▶ Homemade Breakfast Sausage, Three Ways

Mango Blast Smoothie

SERVES 4

▶ *CALORIES PER SERVING* **78** // *SODIUM PER SERVING* **1.25MG**

Portable, light, and satisfying, Mango Blast Smoothie will provide the nutrients and energy needed to power the body until lunchtime. Keep some bananas in the freezer to add to smoothies anytime; to freeze them, peel and place on a tray or pan in the freezer. Once frozen, transfer them to a large sealable plastic bag for longer storage.

2 ripe mangos, peeled and coarsely chopped
2 frozen bananas, coarsely chopped
½ cup nonfat vanilla yogurt
Juice of 1 lime
Ice cubes, if desired
Mint sprigs, for garnish (optional)

1. Place the mangos and bananas in a food processor or blender. Pulse for several seconds to chop and mix the fruit.

2. Add the yogurt and lime juice and process until smooth. If the smoothie isn't thin or cold enough, add a couple of ice cubes and process again until smooth. Garnish with mint sprigs, if desired, and serve immediately.

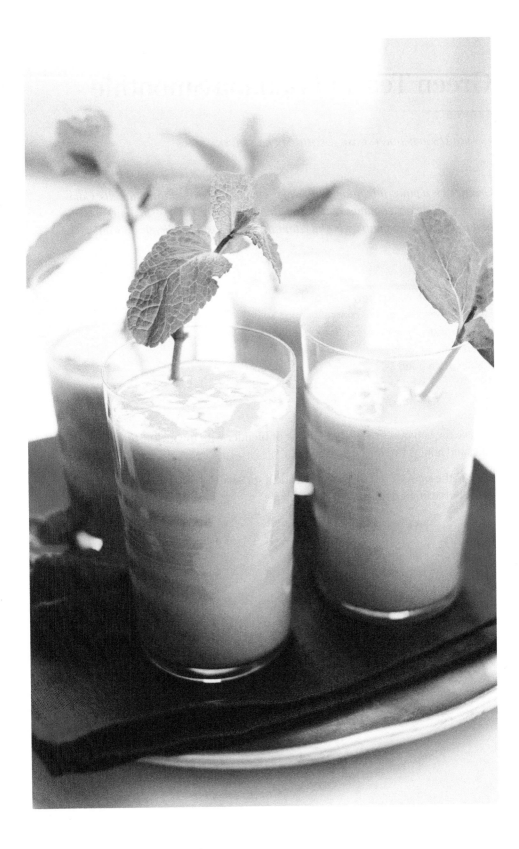

Green Tea and Banana Smoothie

SERVES 2

▶ *CALORIES PER SERVING* **116** // *SODIUM PER SERVING* **38MG**

Green tea is a powerful antioxidant, which cleans and protects human cells. Combine it with melon, bananas, honey, and almond milk for the best-tasting smoothie that is also so rich in nutrients and vitamins, it's almost a medicine, only much more delicious.

2 frozen bananas, coarsely chopped

1 large honeydew melon, coarsely chopped

1 cup strongly brewed green tea (made with 2 teabags), at room temperature

½ cup almond milk

1 tablespoon honey

Freshly squeezed lemon juice, if desired

1. Place the bananas in a food processor or blender with the melon, tea, almond milk, and honey. Process until smooth.

2. Taste the smoothie: if it's too sweet, add a splash of lemon juice and process again. Serve immediately.

The Stomach Soother Smoothie

SERVES 4

▸ *CALORIES PER SERVING* **77** // *SODIUM PER SERVING* **37MG**

Ginger and easy-going-down vanilla yogurt make this a good "morning after" choice or just a soothingly cool, healthy drink to begin the day. Ginger aids in digestion and reduces inflammation in the muscles and joints.

1 frozen banana, coarsely chopped
12 ounces nonfat vanilla yogurt
1 tablespoon honey
1 tablespoon chopped fresh ginger
Ice cubes, if desired
Freshly squeezed lemon juice, if desired

1. Place the banana in a food processor or blender and pulse for several seconds. Add the yogurt, honey, and ginger, and process until smooth, about 1 minute. If the smoothie isn't thin or cold enough, add a couple of ice cubes and process again.

2. Taste the smoothie: if it's too sweet, add a splash of lemon juice and process again. Serve immediately.

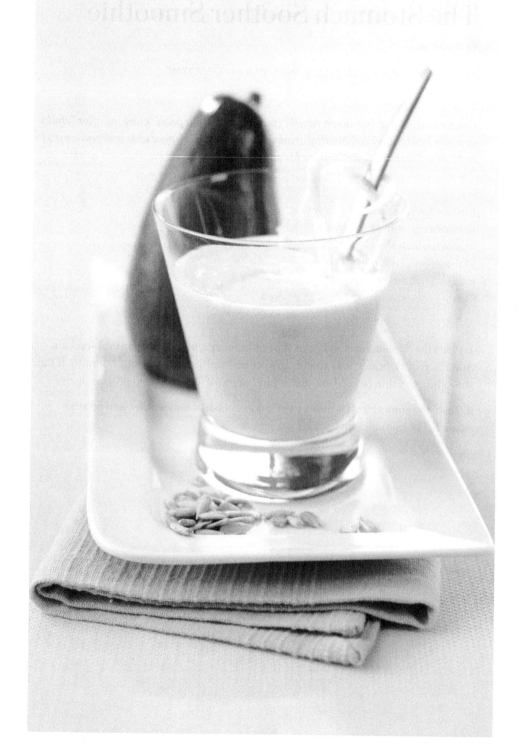

The Green Monster

SERVES 4

▸ *CALORIES PER SERVING* **116** // *SODIUM PER SERVING* **22MG**

Named for the back wall at Fenway Park in Boston, the Green Monster is the kind of smoothie a ball player needs to hit it out of the park. Avocado, apple, and kale make this cold drink taste of tangy fresh greens with hints of sweetness. The knockout power of these ingredients will really amp up your strength in the morning.

2 cups stemmed and coarsely chopped kale leaves
1 Hass avocado, pitted and coarsely chopped
1 apple, peeled and coarsely chopped
½ cup unsweetened apple juice
2 tablespoons freshly squeezed lemon juice
2 or 3 ice cubes

1. Place the kale, avocado, and apple in a food processor or blender and process until smooth. Add the apple juice, lemon juice, and ice and process again. Serve immediately.

Peach Berry Fizz

SERVES 2

▶ *CALORIES PER SERVING* **108** // *SODIUM PER SERVING* **1MG**

Imagine it's Monday morning, the temperature is topping out at 90 degrees, and you need a little bit of encouragement to move on with the day. This is it. Sweet with natural sugars and full of nutrients, it's finished with club soda, which makes for a workweek starter reminiscent of bubbles, cool breezes, mimosas, and good times. Flaxseed and chia seeds can be found in most large grocery stores and all health food stores.

2 ripe peaches, peeled

1 cup blueberries

1 cup coarsely chopped strawberries

1 tablespoon flaxseed or chia seeds

3 or 4 ice cubes

16 ounces club soda or sparkling mineral water

1. Place the peaches, blueberries, strawberries, flaxseed, and ice cubes in a blender and blend until smooth.

2. Fill pint glasses halfway with the mixture and top off with the club soda. Serve immediately.

Hollywood Broiled Grapefruit

SERVES 4

▸ *CALORIES PER SERVING* **150** // *SODIUM PER SERVING* **25MG**

Hollywood used to live by the grapefruit diet: follow the low-carb rules, eat all you want, and always have a grapefruit with every meal. Given the number of skinny starlets, it must have worked. DASH loves grapefruit for the flavor, fiber, and vitamins. Whether summoning the spirit of Joan Crawford or just starting the day right, grapefruit is an excellent choice.

2 grapefruits, halved
2 tablespoons honey, plus more for drizzling
½ cup nonfat vanilla yogurt
1 cup pitted bing cherries
2 tablespoons fresh tarragon leaves

1. Preheat the broiler.

2. Use a serrated knife to loosen the white pith between the grapefruit sections. Scoop out the white pith in the center.

3. Drizzle ½ tablespoon honey over each grapefruit half. Place the grapefruits cut-side up on a baking sheet and broil until the tops are bubbling with juices.

4. Place each grapefruit in a small bowl or on a small plate. Top each with a dollop of vanilla yogurt in the center and ¼ cup cherries; drizzle with additional honey and garnish with ½ tablespoon tarragon leaves. Serve immediately.

Yogurt and Tropical Fruit Parfaits

SERVES 4

▶ *CALORIES PER SERVING* **207** // *SODIUM PER SERVING* **77MG**

Make breakfast parfaits year-round by relying on seasonal fruits paired with companionable ingredients. In the fall, apples, cranberries, and walnuts; in the winter, grapefruit and blood orange; and in the spring, strawberries and rhubarb. Use tall clear glasses to show off the colorful layers and serve with long-handled spoons.

32 ounces nonfat vanilla Greek yogurt
1 mango, peeled and sliced
1 papaya, peeled, seeded, and sliced
2 bananas, sliced
¼ cup unsweetened coconut flakes, toasted

1. Line up 4 tall glasses and fill the bottom of each glass with a large dollop of yogurt. Add a layer of mango and papaya to each glass. Add another layer of yogurt, then a layer of banana, and then sprinkle with coconut.

2. Add another layer of yogurt, and then sprinkle with coconut. Serve immediately.

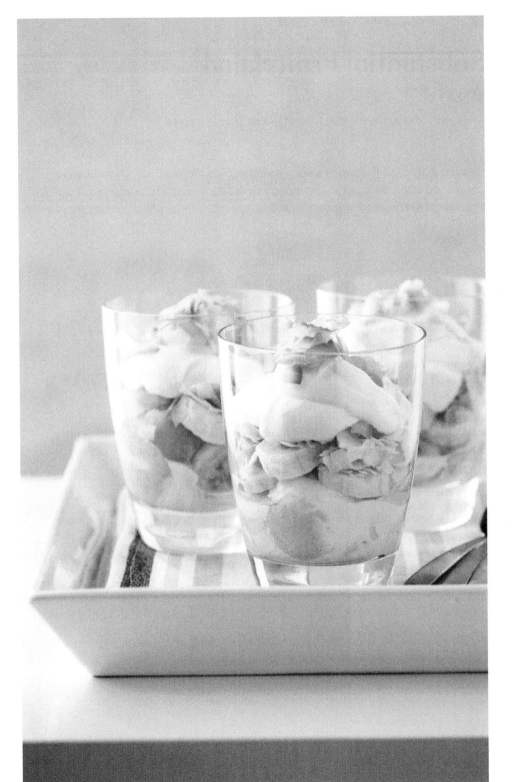

Substantial Fruit Salad

SERVES 4

▶ *CALORIES PER SERVING* **224** // *SODIUM PER SERVING* **29MG**

Avocado makes this fruit salad more substantial than the usual mix of morning berries. Served with a dollop of yogurt mixed with a little honey, this breakfast will make your energy level soar throughout the morning.

2 large Hass avocados, diced

2 fresh peaches, peeled and diced

1 cup diced fresh pineapple

½ red onion, chopped

2–4 tablespoons freshly squeezed lemon or lime juice

Freshly ground pepper

1 cup nonfat plain yogurt

3 tablespoons honey

1. Put the avocados, peaches, pineapple, and onion in a large bowl and mix gently. Add a little bit of the lemon juice, tasting as you go for the right balance of sweet and sour. Season with pepper.

2. In a small bowl, combine the yogurt and honey.

3. Divide the fruit salad among 4 bowls and serve the sweetened yogurt on the side.

Oatmeal with Pistachios and Currants

SERVES 4

▶ *CALORIES PER SERVING* **348** // *SODIUM PER SERVING* **175MG**

Use this as your basic oatmeal recipe and adjust it up or down. Vary it with any of your favorites: sunflower seeds, dried cranberries, raisins, blueberries, strawberries, fresh herbs, pumpkin seeds, raspberries, cashews, walnuts, blackberries, mango chunks, and on and on.

2 cups rolled oats

2 tablespoons honey

2 tablespoons wheat germ, flaxseed oil, or chia seeds

½ cup currants

½ cup pistachios

1 cup soy milk, divided

1. Bring 4 cups water to a boil in a medium saucepan. Stir in the oats and honey and cook according to the package directions.

2. Once the oatmeal is cooked, stir in the wheat germ.

3. Divide the oatmeal among 4 bowls. Top with 2 tablespoons each of currants and pistachios; then pour on ½ cup soy milk. Serve immediately.

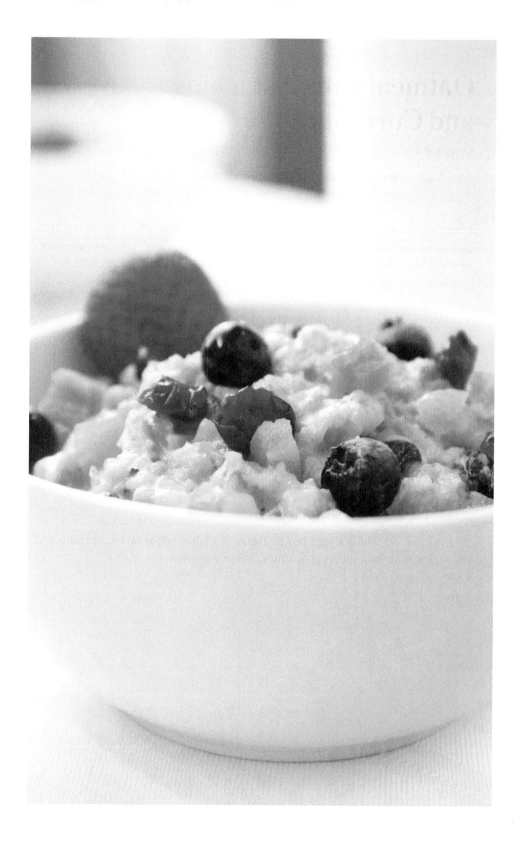

Sweet Potato Oatmeal

SERVES 4

▶ *CALORIES PER SERVING* **388**
▶ *SODIUM PER SERVING* **107MG**

The effects of oatmeal on circulatory health are well known. Add to it a super food like sweet potato, and while there's no guarantee you'll be able to leap a building in a single bound, you might feel inspired to take the stairs.

1 large sweet potato, peeled and diced
4 cups water
2 cups rolled oats
2 tablespoons honey
2 tablespoons wheat germ or chia seeds
4 strawberries, halved or quartered
¼ cup fresh blueberries
¼ cup raisins
¼ cup dried cranberries

1. Place the sweet potato in a medium saucepan and cover with water. Bring to a boil over medium-high heat and cook until tender, about 5 minutes. Drain.

2. Bring the 4 cups of water to a boil in a medium saucepan. Stir in the oats and honey and cook according to package directions.

3. Once the oatmeal is cooked, stir in the wheat germ (or chia seeds) and all but ¼ cup of the sweet potato. Return to the heat and warm through.

4. Divide the oatmeal among 4 bowls. Top with the fresh and dried fruit and the remaining sweet potato, dividing equally, and serve immediately.

Granola, Your Way

SERVES 6

▸ *CALORIES PER SERVING* **559** // *SODIUM PER SERVING* **6MG**

In the 1960s, scientist discovered that the fiber in oats—beta glucan—is special and lowers cholesterol by as much as 23 percent. This granola is a great breakfast for those following a heart-healthy diet. Experiment with other ingredients you like: shredded coconut, flaxseed or chia seeds, or chopped dried apricots or mangos.

4 cups rolled oats

⅓ cup honey

¼ cup canola oil

2 teaspoons vanilla extract

1 teaspoon ground cinnamon

1 cup mixed dried fruit

1 cup chopped mixed nuts or seeds, such as walnuts, cashews, pecans, or sunflower seeds

1. Preheat the oven to 300° F.

2. In a large bowl, combine the oats, honey, oil, vanilla, and cinnamon. Spread evenly on a large rimmed baking sheet.

3. Bake for 15 minutes. Stir the oats well, and then bake for another 15 minutes, or until evenly toasted. Let cool to room temperature.

4. Transfer the granola to a large bowl, add the fruit and nuts, and stir thoroughly to combine. Serve immediately or store in an airtight container for up to 2 weeks.

Acorn Squash, Apple, and Peach "Pie"

SERVES 2

▶ *CALORIES PER SERVING* **257** // *SODIUM PER SERVING* **37MG**

This dish has the flavors of a creamy spiced pumpkin pie without the calories. It makes for a hearty fall breakfast, or it can also be served for dessert. It's healthy, easy to make, and keeps in the refrigerator for several days.

½ acorn squash, seeded and cut into large chunks
2 apples, cored and chopped
1 fresh peach, chopped
2 tablespoons honey
1 tablespoon grated fresh ginger
½ teaspoon ground cinnamon
¼ teaspoon ground nutmeg
Pinch of ground cloves
½ cup low-fat peach yogurt

1. Place the squash in a medium stockpot with water to a depth of 2 inches. Cover and cook over medium-high heat for about 10 minutes, until nearly tender. Cook for a few minutes longer if needed.

2. Add or remove water to bring the depth to about 1 inch. Reduce the heat to medium-low. Add the apples and peaches to the pan, then cover and cook for 5 minutes. Check the squash again; it should be tender and easily pierced with a fork. Continue cooking until it's very tender, being sure to maintain a bit of water in the pan.

3. When the squash is tender, use a fork or tongs to transfer it to a large mixing bowl. Remove the skin with a paring knife and discard. Mash the squash well.

4. Use a slotted spoon to transfer the other fruit from the pot and combine it with the squash. Stir in the honey, ginger, cinnamon, nutmeg, and cloves. Stir well to combine, cover the bowl, and chill in the refrigerator for 1–2 hours. Stir in the yogurt just before serving.

Folded French Omelet

SERVES 4

▶ *CALORIES PER SERVING* **240** // *SODIUM PER SERVING* **132MG**

Leave it to the French to elevate a simple omelet to utter sophistication. Invest in an 8- or 9-inch nonstick frying or omelet pan and experiment until it feels comfortable. It will take practice, but learning how to make a perfect omelet is a skill worth mastering. This recipe calls for bell pepper, but there's a range of vegetables to choose from. Use cheese sparingly for flavor and velvety texture.

Cooking spray
1 cup finely diced green bell pepper
8 large eggs
2 slices low-sodium Swiss cheese
Freshly ground pepper

1. Thinly coat a nonstick skillet with cooking spray and place over medium heat. Add the bell pepper and sauté, stirring frequently, until softened. Transfer to a plate or bowl.

2. Meanwhile, crack the eggs into a large bowl. Beat with a fork until just combined. Do not overbeat and do not add any liquid. There should be no frothy bubbles.

3. Spray the pan again as needed and increase the heat to medium-high. Once hot, pour the eggs into the pan. Using a fork or spatula, stir the eggs frequently as they begin to set. Pull the cooked egg away from the pan's edge and tilt the pan to allow uncooked egg to spread around the edges and set.

4. When the omelet is almost cooked through, spread the bell pepper on the half opposite the handle. Lay the cheese on top. Season with pepper.

5. To fold the omelet, tilt the pan up and away from you, using the fork to loosen the half nearest to the handle. Gently fold the omelet in half over the stuffing. Slide the omelet carefully onto a plate. Cut into quarters and serve immediately.

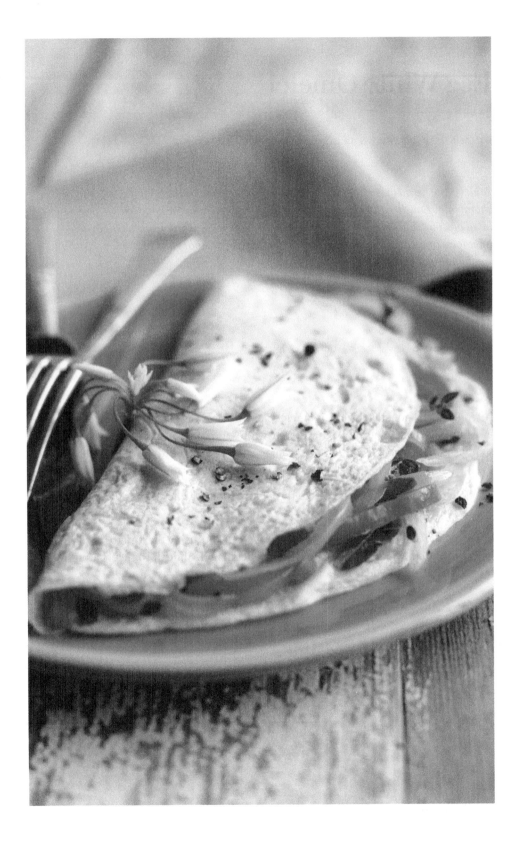

Egg White Omelet

SERVES 4

▶ *CALORIES PER SERVING 42 // SODIUM PER SERVING 133MG*

Athletes the world over confirm that the egg white omelet is the breakfast of champions. Low in calories and sodium, egg whites sustain the body with a large hit of protein. Additions such as chopped bell peppers, mushrooms, zucchini, tomatoes, and green onions increase flavor and nutritional value. Find the combination you like best.

Cooking spray
12 large egg whites, beaten
¼ cup chopped fresh herbs, such as dill, parsley, or chives
Freshly ground pepper

1. Thinly coat a nonstick frying or omelet pan with cooking spray and place over medium-high heat. Once hot, pour the egg whites into the pan. Using a fork or spatula, pull the cooked whites away from the pan's edge and tilt the pan to allow the uncooked whites to spread around and cook.

2. When the omelet is almost cooked through, sprinkle the herbs over the top and season with pepper.

3. To fold the omelet, tilt the pan up and away from you, using the fork to loosen the half closest to the handle. Gently fold the omelet in half. Slide the omelet carefully onto a plate. Cut into quarters and serve immediately.

Creamy "French" Scrambled Eggs

SERVES 4

▸ *CALORIES PER SERVING* **446** *(WITH CHALLAH);* **376** *(WITH MULTIGRAIN)*
▸ *SODIUM PER SERVING* **376MG** *(WITH CHALLAH);* **311MG** *(WITH MULTIGRAIN)*

Almost like a custard, these eggs are made creamy by cooking them long and slow over boiling water. The addition of vinegar makes the eggs even more tender. These are the eggs Jacqueline Onassis loved, and the Carlyle Hotel still serves them on holidays. The simplicity is stunning. Serve with toast points.

8 large eggs
¼ cup low-fat milk
1 tablespoon white vinegar
1 tablespoon unsalted buttery spread
Freshly ground pepper
4 thin slices challah or sprouted no-salt multigrain bread, toasted and cut diagonally

1. Fill the bottom of a double boiler halfway with water and place over medium-high heat. Alternatively, you can set one pan into a slightly larger one to create a double boiler, provided that the base of the top pan doesn't touch the boiling water.

2. Crack the eggs into a large bowl. Add the milk and vinegar and whisk until frothy.

3. Reduce the heat to maintain a gentle simmer. Add the buttery spread to the pan, and when it's just melted, pour in the eggs.

4. Using a wooden spoon, stir the eggs every minute or so as they begin to set. You will need to watch carefully and stir frequently near the end of cooking. The eggs are ready when they have a moist sheen on the outside but are cooked through, about 20 minutes.

5. Divide the eggs among 4 plates and nestle 2 toast points on either side. Serve immediately, garnished with pepper.

Spanish-Style Scrambled Eggs

SERVES 4

▶ *CALORIES PER SERVING* **253** // *SODIUM PER SERVING* **380MG**

Scrambled eggs are yet another ideal canvas for exploring flavors, colors, and textures. Traditionally, Spanish scrambled eggs feature potatoes and pork, but to keep the sodium levels reasonable and make the dish healthier, we've used vegetables instead. The diced bell pepper makes this a little less Spanish but a lot more nutritious.

3 tablespoons extra-virgin olive oil
1 small Spanish onion, diced
¼ cup diced red or green bell pepper
2 garlic cloves, chopped
8 large eggs
¼ cup low-fat milk
Freshly ground pepper

1. Heat the oil in a large skillet over medium-high heat. When the oil is hot, add the onion, bell pepper, and garlic, and sauté for 5 minutes, or until the vegetables are softened. Spread the vegetables evenly across the bottom of the pan.

2. Crack the eggs into a large bowl, add the milk, and beat until frothy. Pour the eggs over the vegetables in the pan. Cook until the eggs are set, about 5 minutes. Season with pepper and serve immediately.

Baked Eggs with Truffle Oil and Fontina Cheese

SERVES 6

▶ *CALORIES PER SERVING* **297** // *SODIUM PER SERVING* **342MG**

These eggs are baked in a muffin tin and slide onto English muffin halves for a lovely presentation. The cheese adds velvety texture, and a little splash of truffle oil flavors the eggs with a royal touch. This is perfect breakfast fare for a crowd. Make sure the muffin tin is nestled securely in a larger pan of water; this water bath is the key to a perfectly tender cooked egg.

Cooking spray

12 large eggs

12 (1 x 1-inch) cubes Fontina cheese

Truffle oil

6 whole-wheat English muffins, split and toasted

1. Preheat the oven to 350° F.

2. Thinly coat a muffin pan with cooking spray. Crack 1 egg into each muffin cup. Put 1 cube of cheese on top of each egg and drizzle with a few drops of truffle oil (a little goes a long way).

3. Position the muffin pan in a larger baking pan filled with 1–2 inches of water. This will ensure even cooking and tender eggs. Carefully slide the pans into the oven and bake for 12–14 minutes, or until the egg whites are firm but the yolks are still runny.

4. Using a thin spatula, remove the eggs from the muffin cups and place 1 egg on each English muffin half. Serve immediately.

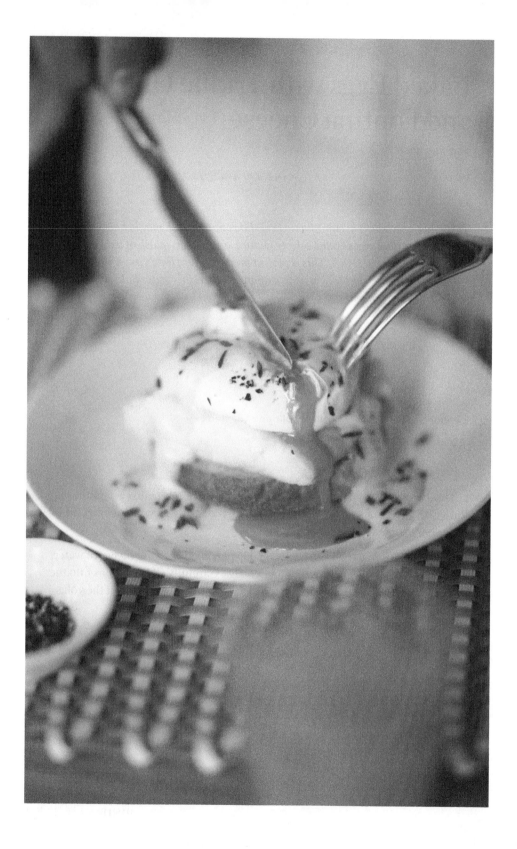

Perfect Poached Eggs
with Lemon Sauce

SERVES 4

▶ *CALORIES PER SERVING* **159** // *SODIUM PER SERVING* **537MG**

This recipe uses the traditional method for poaching a perfect egg. Don't buy a special pot designed just for poaching—the eggs come out looking industrial rather than delectable. You simply need a large skillet, a watchful eye, and a spoon, preferably slotted. The sodium in this dish comes mostly from the whole-wheat bread. To avoid it, serve the eggs atop piles of steamed spinach or use a good sodium-free bread such as the one available from Trader Joe's grocery stores.

For the eggs:
4 large eggs
2 teaspoons apple cider vinegar or unseasoned rice vinegar

For the lemon sauce:
½ cup reduced-sodium chicken broth
2 tablespoons freshly squeezed lemon juice
2 ounces fat-free cream cheese, cut into cubes

To serve:
4 slices whole-wheat bread, toasted
2 tablespoons chopped parsley leaves

To prepare the eggs:

1. Fill a skillet with water to a depth of 1½ inches. Add the vinegar and bring to a simmer over medium-high heat (do not let it boil). Reduce the heat to medium.

2. Crack an egg into a tiny bowl or coffee cup. Carefully slide the egg into the water. Use a spoon to swirl the white tendrils back toward the egg. It should resemble a small pouch in the water. Repeat with the remaining eggs.

3. Cover the pan, turn off the heat, and let the eggs sit in the hot water for 4 minutes. Transfer the eggs with a slotted spoon to paper towels to drain.

continued ▶

To prepare the sauce:

1. In a small saucepan over medium-high heat, whisk together the chicken broth and lemon juice. Simmer for about 3 minutes, or until the liquid is reduced by half. Add the cream cheese and whisk constantly until it melts, about 1 minute.

2. To serve, place a poached egg on each slice of bread. Spoon the lemon sauce over the top and sprinkle with the parsley. Serve immediately.

Easy Breakfast Casserole with Vegetables

SERVES 6

▶ *CALORIES PER SERVING* **400** // *SODIUM PER SERVING* **601MG**

One of the easiest ways to feed a family in the morning, the breakfast casserole is easy for you as well. Add whatever vegetable combinations appeal to you, as this recipe is infinitely adaptable. Here, broccoli and bell pepper were chosen for their amazing nutritional power.

12 large eggs
1 cup nonfat cottage cheese
1 cup nonfat ricotta cheese
Cooking spray
1 cup thinly sliced red bell pepper
1 cup broccoli florets
½ cup cubed reduced-fat cheddar cheese
¼ cup chopped fresh parsley
Freshly ground black pepper

1. Preheat the oven to 350° F. Thinly coat a baking dish with cooking spray.

2. Beat the eggs in a large bowl. Add the cottage cheese and ricotta cheese, and mix thoroughly.

3. Thinly coat a skillet with cooking spray and place over medium-high heat. Once hot, add the bell pepper and broccoli and sauté for 3 to 5 minutes, or until the vegetables are bright in color and just softened.

4. Pour half of the egg mixture into the prepared baking dish. Layer the vegetables over the top, sprinkle with the cheddar and parsley, and then cover with the remaining egg mixture. Season to taste with pepper.

5. Bake in the preheated oven for 45–60 minutes, or until the eggs are set. Let the casserole sit for 5 minutes, then serve.

Crustless Spinach Quiche

SERVES 6

▶ *CALORIES PER SERVING* **333** // *SODIUM PER SERVING* **284MG**

Spinach is a super food. Try and tuck it in anywhere you can: salads, eggs, and sandwiches. Here it's used in a quiche without a crust—and you won't even miss it.

Cooking spray
1 (10-ounce) package frozen chopped spinach, thawed
1 tablespoon canola oil
1 onion, diced
6 large eggs, beaten
1 cup shredded Gruyère
1 teaspoon ground cloves

1. Preheat the oven to 350° F. Thinly coat a pie dish with cooking spray

2. Place the spinach in a colander and squeeze as much water out of it as you can. Press with paper towels to absorb the released water as needed.

3. Heat the oil in a large skillet over medium-high heat. When hot, add the onion and cook until soft and slightly translucent, about 5 minutes. Add the spinach and cook off any released liquid, stirring frequently. Transfer the mixture to the prepared pie dish, spreading it evenly across the bottom.

4. In a medium bowl, beat the eggs. Add the Gruyère and cloves and stir well to incorporate. Pour the eggs over the spinach.

5. Bake for 30 minutes, or until the eggs are set. Let the quiche sit for 5 minutes, then cut into wedges and serve.

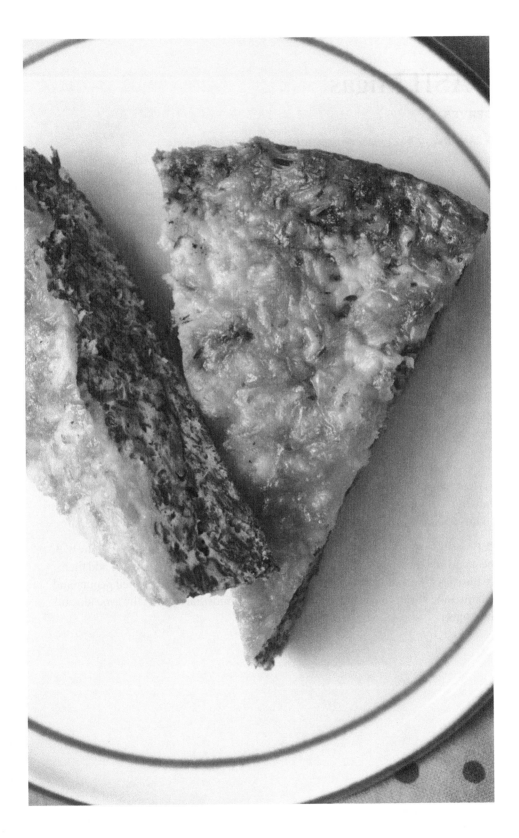

DASH Migas

SERVES 4

▶ *CALORIES PER SERVING* **341** // *SODIUM PER SERVING* **244MG**

If you're raised in a state along the Mexican border, migas are always on the menu. Simply corn tortillas made crisp in a little oil with eggs poured over the top, migas can handle as many additions as you want to throw in. Chorizo, Italian sausage, chicken, cheese, jalapeños, ham, and vegetables are all popular choices. Serving avocado slices on the side offers a good dose of potassium, and the bell pepper and fresh cilantro in the migas provide vitamin C.

2 to 3 tablespoons canola oil
12 (6-inch) corn tortillas
6 large eggs
½ cup diced green bell pepper
¼ cup fresh cilantro leaves
1 avocado, quartered
Hot sauce, for serving

1. Heat the oil in a medium skillet over high heat. Using tongs, slip a corn tortilla into the oil, flipping until it becomes crunchy. Repeat for all the tortillas, adding more canola oil as needed. Set the crisp tortillas aside on paper towels to drain.

2. Break the eggs into a large bowl and beat well. Return the skillet to medium-high heat and add the eggs. Break the tortillas into large bite-sized pieces and add them to the eggs. Continue stirring until the eggs just start to set. Add the bell pepper and cilantro and stir until the eggs are just set. Serve immediately with the avocado and hot sauce.

Grits and Eggs

SERVES 4

▶ *CALORIES PER SERVING* **337** // *SODIUM PER SERVING* **237MG**

Who said comfort food should be reserved for lunch and dinner? Grits is a traditional southern favorite spreading in popularity across the country. Paired with eggs, this dish is a healthful way to start your day with a hearty meal prepared in less than 20 minutes.

1 cup grits
Cooking spray
4 large eggs
1 tablespoon margarine
½ cup reduced-fat cheddar cheese
Freshly ground pepper

1. Bring 3 cups water to a gentle simmer in a medium saucepan over medium heat. Slowly whisk in the grits and cook for 10–15 minutes, stirring frequently.

2. Meanwhile, thinly coat a skillet with cooking spray and cook the 4 eggs sunny-side up or over-easy, as desired.

3. Remove the grits from the heat and stir in the margarine and cheese until melted and well incorporated. Season with pepper. Divide the grits among 4 plates or shallow bowls and top with an egg. Season with pepper and serve.

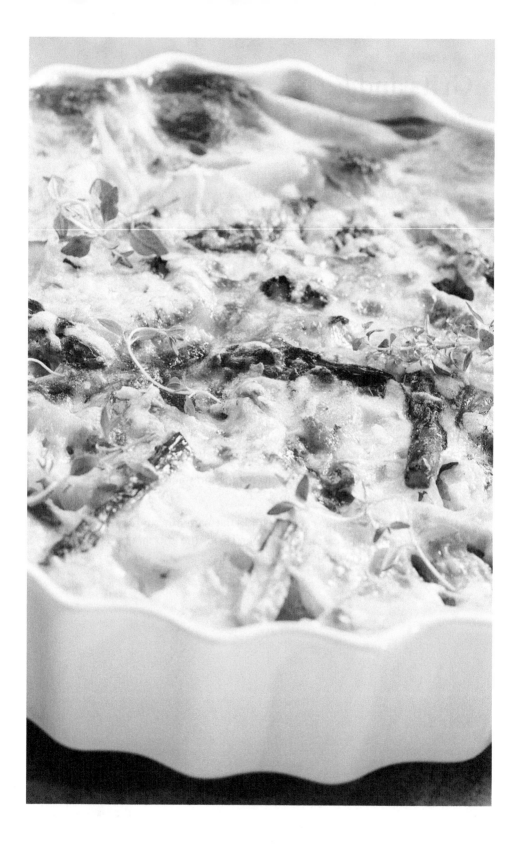

Egg Tart with Sweet Potato Crust

SERVES 4

▶ *CALORIES PER SERVING* **408** // *SODIUM PER SERVING* **282MG**

Shredded sweet potato is filled with eggs, cheese, bell pepper, and onion and baked in a pie dish. The laborious work here is simply shredding the potatoes. Use the real thing, not commercial hash browns.

4 cups shredded sweet potatoes
Cooking spray
½ cup diced onion
½ cup chopped red, green, or yellow bell pepper
1 pound slender asparagus spears, trimmed
6 large eggs
½ cup soy milk
½ cup shredded low-fat cheddar cheese
1 tomato, thinly sliced
Freshly ground pepper

1. Spread the shredded potatoes across several layers of paper towels. Place additional paper towels on top and press firmly to remove as much moisture as possible. Replace with new layers of paper towels and let the sweet potatoes sit for at least 1–2 hours. The drier they are, the better the dish will be.

2. Preheat the oven to 425° F. Thinly coat a pie dish with cooking spray.

3. Press the sweet potatoes evenly into the prepared pie dish to form the crust. (The bottom of a glass is a good tool for pressing them down.) Bake for 25–30 minutes, or until the sweet potatoes become a crunchy brown crust.

4. Thinly coat a small skillet with cooking spray and sauté the onion and bell pepper until just soft. Set aside.

continued ▶

5. In a large bowl, beat the eggs and soy milk together. Stir in the vegetables and cheese.

6. Pour the egg mixture into the crust. Arrange the tomato slices in a pattern on top of the filling. Bake the tart for 25–30 minutes, or until the filling is puffy and golden brown. Serve immediately, garnished with pepper.

Strawberry and Cream Cheese Cakes

SERVES 4

▶ *CALORIES PER SERVING* **145** // *SODIUM PER SERVING* **21MG**

Cream cheese and strawberries are the dominant flavors here, so the humble rice cake is just fine as a base of operations. Pile the cream cheese high with strawberries—or blackberries, raspberries, or blueberries—and fresh basil, and don't feel the slightest bit guilty about enjoying this lucious-tasting breakfast.

½ cup low-fat whipped cream cheese, at room temperature

2 tablespoons honey

2 tablespoons shredded or chopped fresh basil

1 teaspoon lemon zest

1 pint strawberries, hulled and sliced

4 lightly salted rice cakes

4 basil leaves, for garnish

Extra-virgin olive oil, for drizzling

1. Put the cream cheese in a small bowl, and stir in the honey, shredded basil, and lemon zest until thoroughly incorporated.

2. Place the rice cakes on 4 small plates. Spread a few tablespoons of the cream cheese mixture on each rice cake; then divide the strawberries evenly and pile them on top. Garnish with a basil leaf and drizzle with a little oil. Serve immediately.

Cucumber and Ricotta Open-Face Sandwiches

SERVES 4

▸ *CALORIES PER SERVING* **147** // *SODIUM PER SERVING* **330MG**

Few things are easier to grab on the go than a piece of toast slathered with low-fat ricotta and fresh vegetables and herbs. Cut the toast into small squares and this sandwich turns into an appetizer or accompanies a main dish salad or soup. Add any flavor combinations you like: tomato and fresh basil or eggplant and oregano are just two possibilities.

1 cup low-fat ricotta cheese

Zest of ½ lemon

4 slices ciabatta bread, toasted

1 cucumber, thinly sliced

Extra-virgin olive oil, for drizzling

Chopped fresh dill

1. Mix the ricotta and lemon zest in a small bowl. Spread ¼ cup of the ricotta on each piece of toast and pile high with cucumber. Drizzle with a little oil and sprinkle dill over the top. Serve immediately.

Hummus and Sardines on Toast

SERVES 4

▸ *CALORIES PER SERVING* **156** // *SODIUM PER SERVING* **276MG**

In many parts of Scandinavia, fish is a big part of breakfast. The smaller the fish, the healthier it is for you, as there will be less heavy metal in it. Just a few ounces of sardines contain 50 percent of your daily calcium requirement. Add chickpea power in the form of hummus, and this is a fantastic start to the day.

4 slices ciabatta bread, toasted
1 clove garlic, halved
1 cup store-bought hummus or 1 cup Homemade Hummus (page 209)
2 (4-ounce) cans sardines
Freshly squeezed lemon juice
Freshly ground pepper
½ cup chopped parsley leaves, for garnish

1. Rub each ciabatta slice with the cut side of garlic.

2. Spread a thick layer of hummus on each slice. Arrange 2–3 sardines on each and splash with lemon juice. Season with pepper, garnish with the parsley, and serve.

Breakfast Burrito

SERVES 4

▶ *CALORIES PER SERVING* **293** // *SODIUM PER SERVING* **295MG**

A corn tortilla is the perfect vehicle for scrambled eggs, melted cheese, and salsa. Bell pepper and tomato will take you over the daily vitamin C requirement, and the protein from the eggs and cheese will give you a real boost. This breakfast creates excellent morning mojo.

1 cup diced, roasted new potatoes
¼ cup finely minced cilantro leaves
Juice of 1 lime
Cooking spray
4 small whole-wheat tortillas
8 large eggs
2 tablespoons whole milk
Freshly ground pepper
Hot sauce
¼ cup shredded low-sodium cheddar cheese
1 cup baby spinach leaves

1. In a small bowl, combine the potatoes, cilantro, and lime juice. Stir well and let sit for 30 minutes or so at room temperature to blend the flavors.

2. Thinly coat a large skillet with cooking spray and place over medium-high heat. When the pan is hot, add 1 tortilla at a time, frying one side for 30 seconds, then flipping it over and cooking the other side for 30 seconds. Stack the tortillas in a clean dish towel or wrap them in aluminum foil and place in a warm oven.

3. Thinly coat the same pan with more cooking spray and place over medium heat. Break the eggs in a large bowl. Stir in the milk and season with pepper and hot sauce. Whisk the eggs until frothy. Pour the mixture into the skillet and stir frequently as the eggs set. Remove the pan from the heat.

4. To assemble the burritos, heap scrambled eggs on a tortilla, sprinkle with the cheddar, and top with the potato mixture. Top with spinach, roll up, and serve.

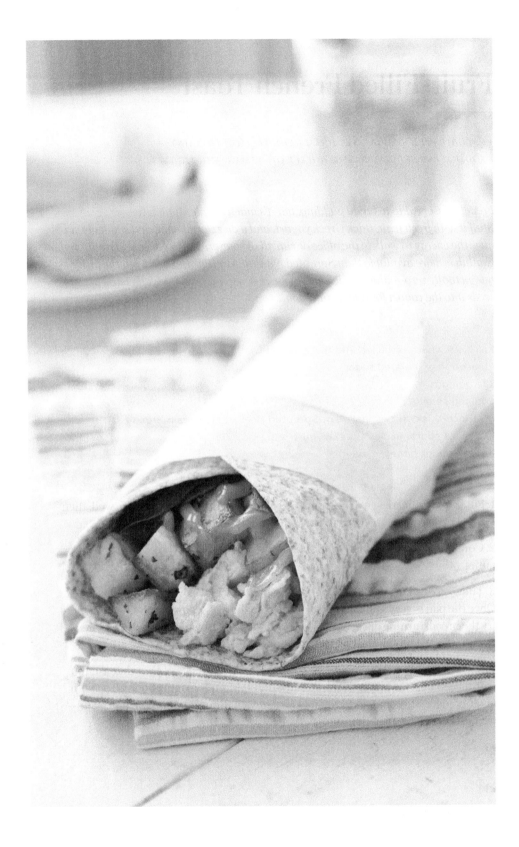

Fruit-Filled French Toast

SERVES 4

▸ *CALORIES PER SERVING* **327** *(CHALLAH);* **317** *(MULTIGRAIN)*
▸ *SODIUM PER SERVING* **248MG** *(CHALLAH);* **173MG** *(MULTIGRAIN)*

French toast is akin to bread pudding, but it's much simpler than its dessert cousin. Stuff it with fresh fruit, thick Greek yogurt, and a drizzle of honey, and suddenly you have the energy to walk to the office or run all of your errands with ease. Traditional challah is more available than Sprouted No-Salt Multigrain Bread, but the latter has virtually zero sodium, which is rare for commercial bread. Mix flaxseed or chia seeds into the yogurt for added nutrition.

....

1 pint strawberries, hulled and thinly sliced
1 teaspoon granulated sugar
3 large eggs
Cooking spray
8 (½-inch-thick) slices challah or Sprouted No-Salt Multigrain Bread
16 ounces nonfat vanilla Greek yogurt
4 tablespoons honey, divided

....

1. Put the strawberries in a medium bowl and stir in the sugar. Combine well; then let the berries macerate for at least 30 minutes.

2. Combine the eggs and 1–2 tablespoons water in a medium bowl. Beat with a fork until frothy.

3. Thinly coat a large skillet with cooking spray and place over medium-high heat. Once the pan is very hot, dip a slice of bread in the egg, let any excess drain off, and fry the bread, turning once, until each side is golden brown. Transfer to a plate and repeat with the remaining bread slices.

4. Spread a few heaping tablespoons of the yogurt on a piece of French toast, top with a layer of strawberries, and drizzle with 1 tablespoon of the honey. Top with another piece of French toast to make a sandwich. Repeat to make 3 more sandwiches. Serve immediately.

Breakfast Hash

SERVES 4

▶ *CALORIES PER SERVING* **329** // *SODIUM PER SERVING* **274MG**

While corned beef is essential to this recipe, it has a huge amount of sodium, so use only a scant cup to add flavor without overdosing on salt. The vegetables here complement the corned beef perfectly, making it a deliciously savory dish.

2–3 tablespoons canola oil
1 cup chopped onion
½ green bell pepper, diced
1 cup shredded corned beef
4 cups diced sweet potatoes
½ cup chopped parsley leaves
Freshly ground pepper

1. Heat 2 tablespoons of the oil in a large skillet over medium-high heat. Add the onion and bell pepper and cook until softened, about 5 minutes.

2. Add the corned beef and potatoes to the pan and stir well. Add the remaining 1 tablespoon of oil if the mixture begins to stick. Using a spatula, press down on the potatoes and hash as it cooks to form a nice crunchy crust.

3. When the bottom of the hash looks evenly browned and crisp, flip it over. Press it down to brown the other side. Continue until the potatoes are cooked through and crisp on the outside.

4. Transfer the hash to a large platter, sprinkle with the parsley, season with pepper, and serve.

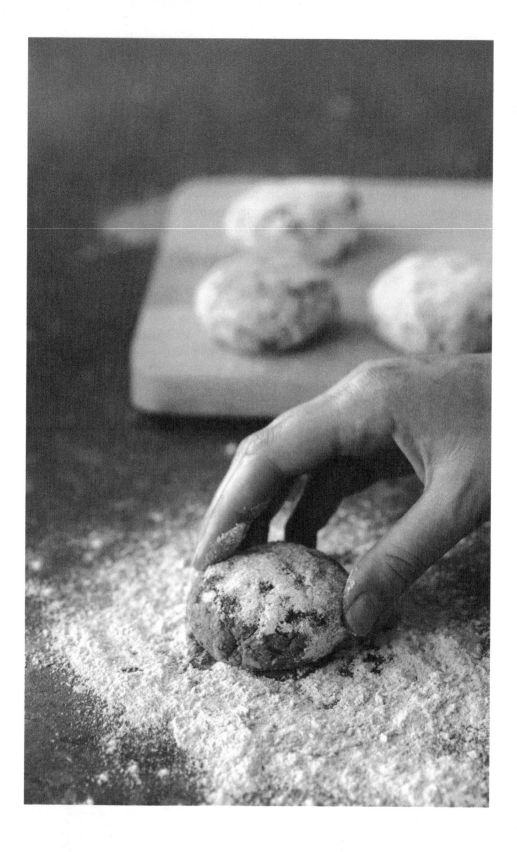

Homemade Breakfast Sausage, Three Ways

SERVES 6

▸ *CALORIES PER SERVING* **330** *(PORK);* **238** *(TURKEY);* **228** *(CHICKEN)*

▸ *SODIUM PER SERVING* **106MG** *(PORK);* **125MG** *(TURKEY);* **109MG** *(CHICKEN)*

Commercially prepared sausages contain an amount of salt that rivals the Dead Sea. You don't have to give up your morning breakfast meats—just make your own version, leave out the salt, and spice it up big. Ground pork, turkey, and chicken are interchangeable here, so try making some of each and pick a favorite. Egg whites add heft and juiciness to your sausage and even more lean protein.

2 pounds ground pork, turkey, or chicken

2 large egg whites, beaten until frothy

2 teaspoons crushed red pepper flakes

1 tablespoon chopped sage

1 tablespoon chopped marjoram

⅛ teaspoon ground cloves

Zest of ½ lemon

Cooking spray

1. In a large bowl, crumble the ground meat. Add the egg whites and knead the mixture with clean hands until the egg is just incorporated into the meat. Do not overmix.

2. Add the red pepper flakes, sage, marjoram, cloves, and lemon zest to the meat mixture and combine thoroughly with your hands. Remove a palm-sized portion of meat from the bowl and form it into a firm, round patty. Set aside on a large plate. Repeat until all of the sausage patties are formed.

3. Thinly coat a large skillet with cooking spray and place it over medium-high heat. Fry the sausages in batches, being sure to leave enough space between them to brown evenly. Serve immediately or place in a warm oven until ready to serve.

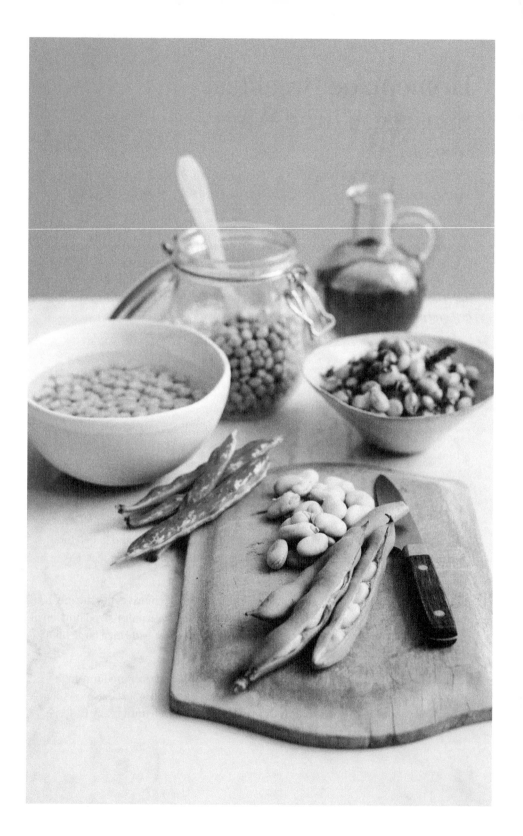

CHAPTER THIRTEEN

DASH Lunches

- Niçoise-Style Salad
- Orange, Avocado, and Shrimp Salad
- Watermelon, Feta, and Mint Summer Salad
- Massaged Kale Salad
- Flattened Chicken on Arugula Salad
- Crunchy Chicken Salad
- White Bean and Sage Soup
- Homemade Tomato Soup
- Melon Soup with Mint and Yogurt
- Cold Avocado and Shrimp Soup
- Vegetable and Mozzarella Frittata
- Vegetable Napoleons
- Almost Mexican Pita
- Vegetable and Hummus Pita
- Wild Salmon Salad Pita
- Roasted Vegetables on Ciabatta

- Quinoa with Vegetables and Toasted Pecans
- Pasta Caprese
- Cold Soba Noodles with Peanut Sauce
- Mini Crab Cakes on Baby Greens
- Simple Rosemary Salmon
- Noodle Salad with Shrimp and Cucumber
- Spicy Chickpeas and Turkey
- Turkey Burgers with Cranberry-Scallion Sauce
- Lightning-Fast Chicken Stir-Fry
- Chicken Curry
- Vietnamese Pork Sandwiches
- Soft Beef Tacos
- Bobotie Lite
- Filet Mignon with Red Wine au Jus

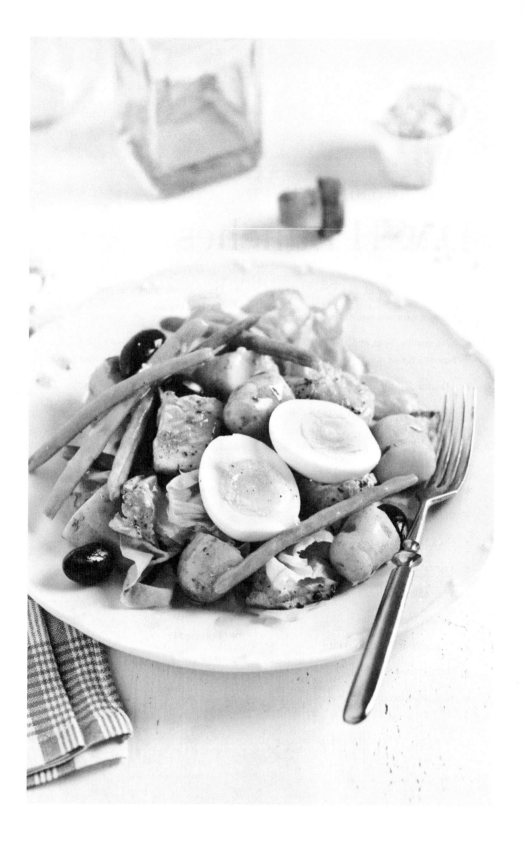

Niçoise-Style Salad

SERVES 6

▶ *CALORIES PER SERVING* **385** // *SODIUM PER SERVING* **448MG**

This classic French salad can be built with a never-ending variety of vegetables, herbs, and vinaigrettes. It rarely tastes the same in any two places. It does, however, traditionally include tuna, hard-boiled eggs, and blanched haricots verts—or their American cousin, green beans. Niçoise makes a bountiful, beautiful presentation arranged on a large platter. Here, thick, meaty slices of Italian tuna in olive oil are called for; don't substitute them—you won't regret it.

For the salad

1 pound small new potatoes

1 pound green beans, ends trimmed

1 head butter lettuce, leaves separated

2 (7-ounce) jars tuna in olive oil (preferably Flott, Callipo, or Wild Planet)

1 yellow bell pepper, sliced into thin strips

1 red bell pepper, sliced into thin strips

1 bunch large radishes, thinly sliced

1 large cucumber, thinly sliced

5 hard-boiled eggs, quartered

For the vinaigrette:

1 clove garlic, minced

3 tablespoons freshly squeezed lemon juice

1 tablespoon Dijon mustard

2 shallots, minced

½ cup extra-virgin olive oil

¼ cup chopped parsley leaves

To make the salad:

1. Boil a large pot of water over high heat. Add the potatoes and cook for about 20 minutes, or until a fork can just pierce the flesh. The potatoes will still be firm; do not overcook. Drain and set aside.

continued ▶

2. Refill the pot with water and return to high heat. Boil the green beans for 2–3 minutes. They should still be a vibrant green and just fork-tender. Run cold water over the beans to stop the cooking process. Drain thoroughly and set aside.

To make the vinaigrette:

1. Put the garlic, lemon juice, mustard, and shallots in a small bowl and whisk thoroughly. Drizzle the olive oil into the bowl in a thin stream, whisking constantly. Stir in the parsley.

2. To assemble the salad, line a large platter with the butter lettuce leaves. Arrange the tuna, potatoes, green beans, bell peppers, radishes, cucumber, and hard-boiled eggs in separate mounds around the platter and drizzle the vinaigrette over all. Serve any extra vinaigrette on the side.

Orange, Avocado, and Shrimp Salad

SERVES 4

▶ *CALORIES PER SERVING* **325** // *SODIUM PER SERVING* **64MG**

With 16 milligrams of fiber, large amounts of vitamin C, and a low sodium content, this composed salad is DASH diet perfection. Colorful and textured, the ingredients are a great midwinter reminder that summer will come again.

1 pound large shell-on shrimp

4 medium navel oranges

2 medium avocados, pitted and thinly sliced

Freshly squeezed lemon juice

5 tablespoons extra-virgin olive oil

3 tablespoons thawed orange juice concentrate

¼ cup cilantro leaves, finely chopped

4 cups butter lettuce, torn into bite-sized pieces

1. Bring a large pot of water to a boil. Add the shrimp (with shells) and cook until just pink, about 3 minutes. Drain and set aside.

2. Peel and section the oranges over a bowl to catch the juice. Set aside.

3. Coat the slices of avocado with lemon juice so they won't turn brown.

4. In a small bowl, whisk together the olive oil, orange juice concentrate, and cilantro.

5. Peel and devein the shrimp.

6. To assemble the salad, divide the butter lettuce among 4 plates. Add a layer of orange sections and then a layer of avocado slices. Pile shrimp in the center of each salad, and then drizzle with the olive oil mixture. Serve.

Watermelon, Feta, and Mint Summer Salad

SERVES 4

▸ *CALORIES PER SERVING* **140** // *SODIUM PER SERVING* **57MG**

In the heat of summer, few dishes create a physical sensation as cooling and juicy as this one. Watermelon has natural sugars and is a powerhouse of vitamins A and C. Feta provides a nice tang to counter the sweet fruit and puts even more A and C on the plate. Mint, filled with potassium, magnesium, and even omega-3 and omega-6 fatty acids, hits the mouth, and suddenly the summer heat loses its teeth. The combination is magical.

2 pounds watermelon, cut into 1-inch pieces

¼ cup feta cheese, coarsely crumbled

1 bunch baby spinach

1 bunch fresh mint leaves, coarsely chopped

Freshly ground black pepper

Extra-virgin olive oil

Freshly squeezed lemon juice (optional)

1. Put the watermelon in a large serving bowl. Add the feta, spinach, and mint. Grind the pepper over the top and add the olive oil to taste.

2. Fold the ingredients together gently so as not to break apart the watermelon and feta chunks, tasting and adding more pepper and olive oil as needed. If desired, add the juice of half a lemon to intensify and brighten the flavors in this dish.

3. Divide the salad among 4 plates, garnish with mint, and serve with a dark, nut-filled bread or basket of whole-grain flatbreads.

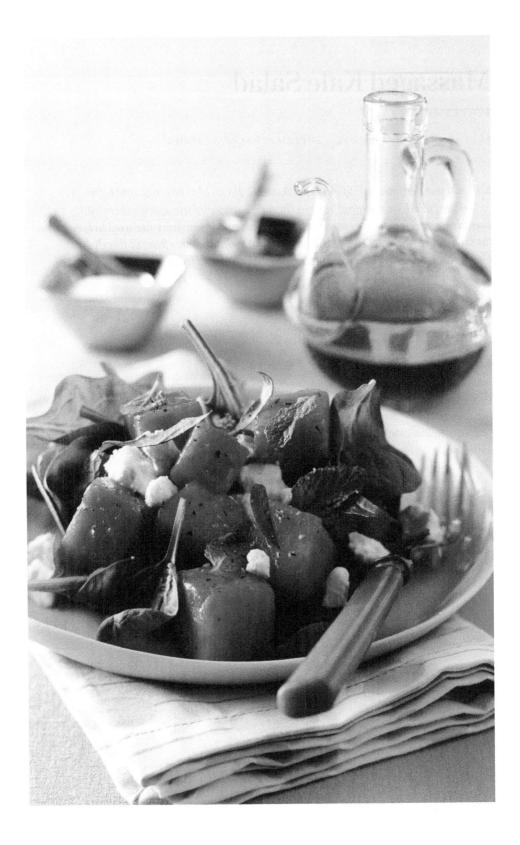

Massaged Kale Salad

SERVES 4

▸ *CALORIES PER SERVING* **262** // *SODIUM PER SERVING* **179MG**

Kale is a wonder food, full of vitamins A and C. It can also be tough and bitter. A technique called "massaging" softens the kale leaves and transforms them into sweet leaves perfect for an entrée salad. Sea salt and lemon juice are used to break the kale down, and that's where the majority of sodium comes from in this dish. Using raw or oven-roasted vegetables, roasted nuts, and fresh or dried fruit really makes this salad sing.

1 bunch kale, stems removed, leaves torn into bite-sized pieces
Freshly squeezed lemon juice
¼ teaspoon fine sea salt
½ cup walnut pieces
½ cup dried cranberries
½ cup shredded carrots
Freshly ground black pepper
Extra-virgin olive oil (optional)

1. Put the kale in a large bowl, squeeze the lemon juice over the top, and add the salt. Using clean hands, massage the kale for 5 minutes, squeezing and kneading it as you would someone's shoulders. The kale will break down and shrink slightly.

2. Add the walnuts, cranberries, and carrots and toss well to combine. Season with pepper to taste. If the salad seems dry, drizzle on a little olive oil and more lemon juice to taste. Serve immediately.

Flattened Chicken on Arugula Salad

SERVES 4

▸ *CALORIES PER SERVING* **345** // *SODIUM PER SERVING* **108MG**

In the United States, the skinless, boneless chicken breast is the most popular cut of chicken to prepare. It's high in lean protein, moderate in calories, and low in fat, making it versatile and appealing. Simple, quick cooking, and satisfying, a flattened chicken breast is perfectly matched here with leafy greens for incomparable nutrition.

4 skinless, boneless chicken breast halves

3 tablespoons margarine

2 shallots, minced

5 ounces arugula

2 tablespoons thyme leaves

2 tablespoons extra-virgin olive oil

2 tablespoons balsamic vinegar

Freshly ground pepper

1. Place the chicken breast halves between two sheets of plastic wrap and pound them to a thickness of ½ to ¾ inches.

2. In a large skillet, melt the margarine. Add the shallots and cook for 1 to 2 minutes. Add the chicken breasts and cook on each side for about 4 minutes, or until lightly browned.

3. Toss the arugula and thyme with the oil and balsamic vinegar, and season with pepper. Divide the salad among 4 plates. Top each with a chicken breast and drizzle with a little of the pan juices. Serve immediately.

Crunchy Chicken Salad

SERVES 4

▶ *CALORIES PER SERVING* **398** // *SODIUM PER SERVING* **269MG**

Crisp fresh vegetables, fruit, nuts, herbs, and chicken are held together with a small amount of mayo and piled atop butter lettuce for a mid-day power punch of protein, vitamins, and fiber.

....

2 whole chicken breasts, split into 2 pieces each
1 cup halved grapes
½ cup cashew pieces
¼ cup raisins
1 small apple, cored and coarsely chopped
1 stalk celery, thinly sliced
¼ cup low-fat mayonnaise
¼ cup shredded basil leaves
4 large butter lettuce leaves
Whole basil leaves, for garnish
Freshly ground pepper, for garnish

....

1. Bring a large pot of water to a boil over medium-high heat. Add the chicken breasts and poach for about 15 minutes, or until the chicken is fully cooked, without any traces of pink. Transfer the chicken to paper towels to drain and let cool completely. You can strain the cooking water and freeze it in an airtight container to use for chicken stock, if desired.

2. Shred the chicken into a large bowl, discarding the skin and bones. Add the grapes, cashews, raisins, apple, celery, mayonnaise, and basil and toss well to combine thoroughly. If the salad is a little dry, add more mayonnaise, 1 tablespoon at a time, until the salad reaches the desired consistency.

3. Place 1 lettuce leaf on each of 4 plates and divide the chicken salad evenly among them. Garnish with a basil leaf and a few grinds of pepper. Serve immediately or chill in the refrigerator for 1 hour, if desired.

White Bean and Sage Soup

SERVES 4

▶ *CALORIES PER SERVING* **311** // *SODIUM PER SERVING* **171MG**

Chicken soup may be good for the soul, but this bean soup is great for the body. Full of fiber, this creamy soup is rich, easy to make, and completely satisfying. Add croutons or crumbled flatbread as a garnish if you crave a little crunch. Be careful, though: people have been known to dream of this hot soup, even in August. Note that you need to plan ahead when making this recipe, as the beans must soak overnight.

1 pound dried cannellini beans
2 tablespoons olive oil
1 onion, chopped
5 fresh sage leaves, coarsely chopped
4 cloves garlic, minced
5 cups low-sodium chicken broth
½ cup heavy cream
Extra-virgin olive oil, for drizzling

1. The night before making the soup, put the beans in a large pot or bowl and cover with water. Let them soak overnight. Drain and set aside.

2. Heat the olive oil in a large pot over medium-high heat. Add the onion, sage, and garlic and cook for 5 minutes, or until the mixture is very fragrant and the onion is soft.

3. Add the chicken broth. Increase the heat to high and bring to a boil. Add the soaked beans, cover, and cook for 30–40 minutes. Check the pot from time to time and add water as needed.

4. Remove the pot from the heat. Once the beans have cooled slightly, process in batches in a food processor until smooth. Return the mixture to the pot over medium heat. Stir in the cream and heat through.

5. Ladle the soup into 4 bowls, drizzle with olive oil, and serve.

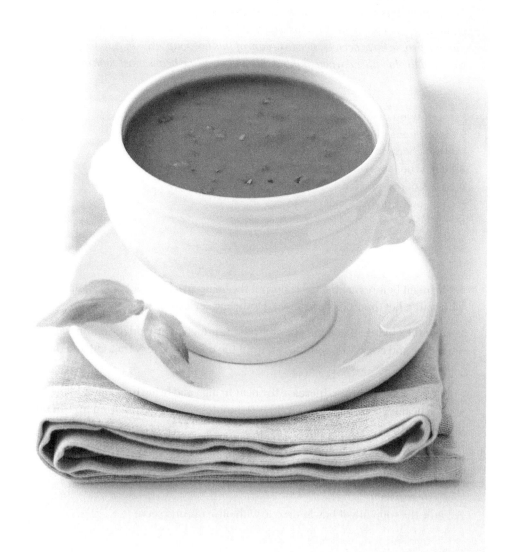

Homemade Tomato Soup

SERVES 6

▸ *CALORIES PER SERVING* **115** // *SODIUM PER SERVING* **190MG**

If you can, make this soup with Roma tomatoes from a farmers' market, but store-bought will work fine, too. This is a simple American classic. You can almost see Mom through the curling steam rising from the hot soup. Serve this with flatbread or thin slices of toasted ciabatta.

3 pounds Roma tomatoes, quartered

2 (14.5-ounce) cans low-sodium, fat-free chicken broth

1 stalk celery, thinly sliced

¼ cup chopped basil leaves

6 ounces nonfat plain Greek yogurt

Whole basil leaves, for garnish

Freshly ground pepper

1. Put the tomatoes, chicken broth, celery, and basil in a large pot and cook over medium-high heat for at least 30 minutes, or until all the tomatoes lose their shape and become soft. Remove the pan from the heat and let the soup cool slightly.

2. Transfer the soup to blender or food processor in two batches or use an immersion blender to puree until smooth and velvety.

3. Return the soup to the pot, if needed, and reheat over medium-low heat. Ladle the soup into bowls and garnish with a generous spoonful of yogurt and a few basil leaves. Season with pepper. The soup can also be chilled and served cold.

Melon Soup with Mint and Yogurt

SERVES 4

▶ *CALORIES PER SERVING* **192** // *SODIUM PER SERVING* **134MG**

This refreshing soup is meant to be eaten ice-cold on a hot day. Don't be fooled by its sweet beauty: it offers a huge load of vitamin C that will support the immune system as well as cleanse and cool the palate. Cantaloupe is used here, but feel free to substitute any favorite melon. Choose your melons with your hands and your nose. They should feel heavy and dense when you pick them up; ripe melons smell sweet. Note that this soup must be prepared the day before serving.

2 large cantaloupes

2 tablespoons freshly squeezed lime juice

2 tablespoons honey

¼ cup ginger ale

½ cup mint leaves

½ cup plain yogurt, plus additional for serving

4–6 mint sprigs, for serving

1. Halve and seed the cantaloupes; then scoop out the flesh and cut it into large chunks.

2. Add the melon, lime juice, honey, ginger ale, mint, and yogurt to a blender or food processor, and process until the mixture is smooth. Transfer to a large bowl, cover, and refrigerate for at least 1 day.

3. Ladle the soup into chilled bowls, and serve with a tiny dollop of yogurt in the center and a mint sprig for garnish.

Cold Avocado and Shrimp Soup

SERVES 4

▸ *CALORIES PER SERVING* **518** // *SODIUM PER SERVING* **189MG**

Green, fresh, and filled with fiber and vitamin C, avocado soup is velvety and smooth. Aside from a three-minute boil for the shrimp, this is a no-cook recipe and thus should be a go-to during hot weather. In the wintertime, all the vibrant green in this soup will have you dreaming of sunlit summer lawns.

2 medium avocados, pitted and roughly chopped
1 cucumber, peeled, seeded, and roughly chopped
½ head romaine lettuce, torn into large pieces
1 teaspoon chopped garlic
1 cup water
Freshly squeezed lemon juice
1 cup coarsely chopped large shrimp
¼ cup coarsely chopped red bell pepper
1 tablespoon finely minced red onion
2 tablespoons freshly squeezed lime juice

1. Put the avocados, cucumber, lettuce, garlic, water, and lemon juice (to taste) in a blender or food processor and process until smooth. Transfer to a large bowl, cover, and refrigerate for at least 1 hour.

2. Meanwhile, bring a small pot of water to a boil. Add the shrimp and cook for 3 minutes, or until opaque. Drain well.

3. Combine the shrimp, bell pepper, onion, and lime juice in a small bowl. Stir well and set aside for 1 hour to let the flavors blend.

4. To serve, divide the shrimp mixture among 4 soup bowls. Ladle the chilled soup over the top and serve immediately.

Vegetable and Mozzarella Frittata

SERVES 4

▶ *CALORIES PER SERVING* **317** // *SODIUM PER SERVING* **218MG**

France has the omelet and Italy has the frittata. The beauty of the frittata is it does not need to be folded, just run under the broiler for a minute or two to firm up the top of the eggs. Like an omelet, a frittata can be stuffed with a huge range of ingredients so feel free to add more vegetables. Served with a salad, this is a wonderful late supper as well.

For the salad:

1 (5-ounce) package mixed greens

½ cup chopped mixed herbs, including parsley, dill, cilantro, thyme, and oregano

Extra-virgin olive oil

Balsamic vinegar

For the frittata:

1–2 tablespoons olive oil, plus more if needed

½ cup green bell pepper, chopped

1 cup chanterelle mushrooms, sliced if large

12 eggs

½ cup chopped basil leaves, chopped

½ cup shredded, reduced-fat mozzarella cheese

Cooking oil spray

To make the salad:

1. Put the mixed greens into a large serving bowl.

2. Clean the herbs, discarding any stems, then chopping finely. Add them to the greens and toss thoroughly to incorporate.

continued ▶

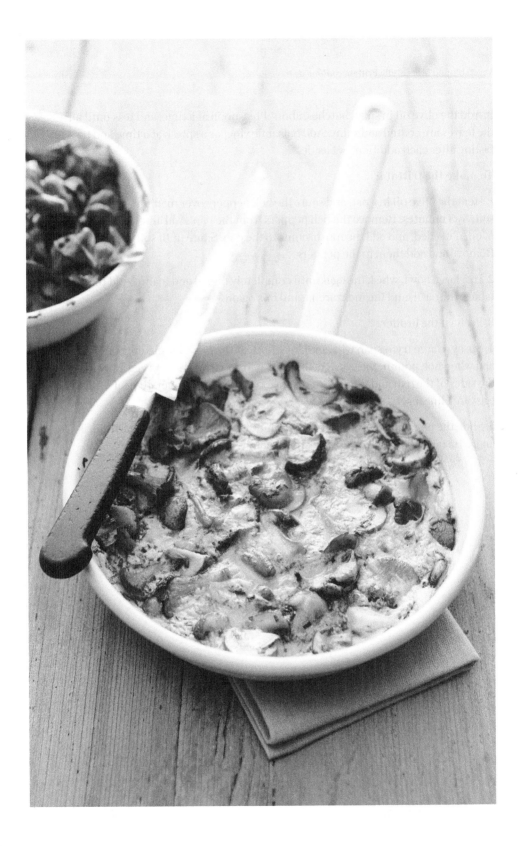

3. Add the olive oil in small batches, about 1 teaspoon at a time, and toss until all the leaves are coated and shiny. Add balsamic vinegar a splash at a time and toss, tasting after each addition. Set aside.

To make the frittata:

1. Heat the olive oil in a pan and sauté the bell peppers over medium-high heat until soft, 3–5 minutes. Remove the bell peppers from the pan. Add another tablespoon of oil, if needed, and add the mushrooms to the pan. Sauté until soft, 5–8 minutes. Remove and add them to the peppers.

2. In a large bowl, whisk the eggs until completely mixed and foamy. Add the vegetables, the basil, and the mozzarella, and mix again.

3. Preheat the broiler.

4. Spray a large frying pan with cooking oil. Heat the pan over medium-high heat, and when hot, pour in the eggs. As they begin to cook, lift the firm egg away from the sides of the pan and tilt it to let the uncooked egg flow under. Repeat until the eggs are almost set.

5. Slide the pan under the broiler for 1–2 minutes, until the top of the frittata is set and is turning golden brown. Serve immediately.

Vegetable Napoleons

SERVES 4

▶ *CALORIES PER SERVING* **305** // *SODIUM PER SERVING* **314MG**

A stack of roasted vegetables sprinkled with feta cheese is a superb, speedy lunch. This is a beautiful, orderly pile of fiber and nutrients that you will be proud to serve even to your most illustrious guests. Serve with thin toasted slices of whole-wheat bread or flatbread to pass at the table.

¼ cup extra-virgin olive oil

2 tablespoons dried oregano

Freshly ground pepper

1 large eggplant, sliced lengthwise into 1-inch-thick slices

1 large zucchini, sliced lengthwise into 1-inch-thick slices

2 large tomatoes, quartered and seeded

½ cup crumbled feta cheese

Raspberry vinegar, for drizzling

½ cup chopped parsley

1. Whisk the olive oil in a small bowl with the oregano and pepper. Using a brush or your fingers, coat all cut sides of the vegetables with the oil mixture. Let sit for at least 1 hour.

2. Preheat the oven to 400° F.

3. Spread the vegetables in a single layer on a rimmed baking sheet—you may need to roast them in batches. Roast for 20 to 30 minutes, or until the vegetables are softened yet still retain their shape.

4. Sprinkle each vegetable slice with a little feta cheese. Return the pan to the oven and cook for 2 to 3 minutes more to let the cheese just melt. Let the vegetables cool to room temperature.

5. To serve, place a slice of eggplant on each of 4 plates. Top with a slice zucchini, then a piece of tomato; continue layering until you have 4 equal stacks. Drizzle each stack with a little raspberry vinegar and sprinkle with parsley. Serve immediately.

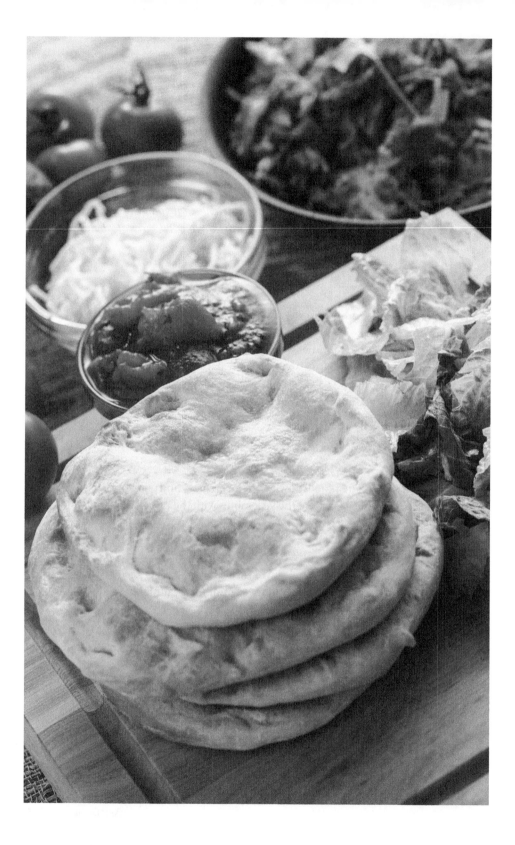

Almost Mexican Pita

SERVES 4

▶ *CALORIES PER SERVING* **324** // *SODIUM PER SERVING* **414MG**

Cumin, chile powder, and salsa give this chicken salad sandwich a decidedly Mexican flavor, but the splash of balsamic vinegar adds a unique dimension and brings the taste of Italy into play. Use leftover roast chicken as a starting point to make this quick and filling lunch.

3 tablespoons olive oil

2 tablespoons balsamic vinegar

1 teaspoon ground cumin

1 teaspoon ground mild chile powder

8 ounces cooked chicken, shredded

2 pita rounds, halved

¼ cup shredded reduced-fat, low-sodium Monterey jack cheese

½ cup prepared salsa, mild or spicy to taste

1 medium tomato, thinly sliced

2 cups chopped romaine lettuce

1. In a large bowl, whisk together the olive oil, vinegar, cumin, and chile powder. Add the shredded chicken and toss well to coat.

2. Tuck the chicken into the pitas, dividing equally. Add the cheese, salsa, tomato, and lettuce. Serve immediately.

Vegetable and Hummus Pita

SERVES 4

▶ *CALORIES PER SERVING* **158** // *SODIUM PER SERVING* **271MG**

Vegetarians worldwide are intimate with salad stuffed in a pita and slathered with lemony hummus. Endlessly versatile, this is an excellent way to pile on the vegetables, get a nice hit of protein, and deliver it all in a pita, which is a much healthier choice than most commercially made breads.

1 cup store-bought hummus or Homemade Hummus (page 209)

¼ cup chopped basil or parsley

1 tablespoon lemon zest

1 tablespoon extra-virgin olive oil

Freshly ground pepper

2 whole-wheat pitas, split

2 cups chopped red leaf, romaine, or butter lettuce

2 medium carrots, shredded

1 cucumber, thinly sliced

1 red onion, thinly sliced

1 large tomato, thinly sliced

1. In a small bowl, stir together the hummus, basil or parsley, lemon zest, and oil. Season with pepper and mix until smooth.

2. Spread a few tablespoons of hummus on the inside of each pita. Tuck some of the lettuce, carrots, cucumber, red onion, and tomato into each pita. Drizzle additional hummus into the center of the vegetables, if desired, and serve.

Wild Salmon Salad Pita

SERVES 4

▸ *CALORIES PER SERVING* **168** // *SODIUM PER SERVING* **295MG**

Forget tuna salad sandwiches—salmon salad is the way to go. Most canned salmon is wild-caught. Oddly, most fresh salmon is farmed. The cost difference between the two is staggering: a large can of wild salmon costs around $4, but a pound of fresh farmed is typically $10 to $18, with fresh wild-caught salmon running even higher. Wild salmon runs in colder, deeper waters, which means less pollution and heavy metal exposure. Salmon has many nutritional benefits over tuna as well: Less sodium, twice the vitamin E, three times the folate, and a full day's supply of vitamin D.

1 (14- to 16-ounce) can wild salmon
¼ cup mayonnaise
1 medium red onion, finely diced
2 tablespoons chopped fresh dill
Zest of 1 lemon
8 large leaves red or green leaf lettuce
2 whole-wheat pitas, split

1. Combine the salmon, mayonnaise, red onion, dill, and lemon zest in a medium bowl and mix well to combine.

2. Tuck 2 lettuce leaves into each pita and put a few heaping tablespoons of salmon salad between them. Serve immediately.

Roasted Vegetables on Ciabatta

SERVES 6

▶ *CALORIES PER SERVING* **333** // *SODIUM PER SERVING* **263MG**

Ciabatta is a white bread with a hard crust that is well suited for an open-faced sandwich of roasted vegetable. Toast the bread lightly, slather it with flavored mayo, and pile on the vegetables. If you can't find a low-sodium chili sauce, be advised that the difference between it and regular is a whopping 200 milligrams of sodium, so you may want to skip it.

1 pound eggplant, peeled, quartered, and cut into long, thin pieces

2 zucchini, thinly sliced

2 red bell peppers, sliced into thin strips

2 tomatoes, quartered

¼ cup extra-virgin olive oil

3 tablespoons chopped fresh oregano or 2 tablespoons dried oregano

Freshly ground black pepper

12 slices ciabatta bread, lightly toasted

Extra-virgin olive oil, for serving

4 tablespoons real mayonnaise, divided

1 tablespoon low-sodium chili sauce

1 tablespoon chopped cilantro

Minced fresh parsley, for serving

1. Preheat oven to 400 degrees F.

2. Put the eggplant, zucchini, bell peppers, and tomatoes in a large mixing bowl. Add the olive oil and oregano, tossing to coat all the vegetables. Season with pepper to taste.

3. Spread the vegetables on a shallow baking pan. Roast for 1 hour, turning the vegetables once after 30 minutes. Let cool. (To store the vegetables for later use, place in large sealable plastic bags or covered bowls with 1–2 tablespoons olive oil to keep them moist. Do not refrigerate.)

4. Put half of the mayonnaise in each of two small bowls. In one bowl, stir in the chili sauce. In the other, stir in the cilantro.

5. Spread half of the bread slices with the chili mayo and the other half with the cilantro mayo. Pile high with vegetables and then finish with a drizzle of extra-virgin olive oil and a dusting of parsley. Serve immediately.

Quinoa with Vegetables and Toasted Pecans

SERVES 4

▶ *CALORIES PER SERVING* **413** // *SODIUM PER SERVING* **307MG**

If quinoa was the fuel that built the Aztec civilization, imagine what it can do for you. Fresh vegetables and herbs weave color throughout this dish, and a simple vinaigrette holds it together. Quinoa is perfect for experimenting with: use this recipe as a starting point and then modify it to try different vegetables, nuts, and dried fruits in whatever combinations please you. This dish will keep in the refrigerator for a day or two, developing even more flavor. Bring it to room temperature, drizzle on a little more olive oil to rehydrate, and serve.

For the quinoa:
2 cups quinoa
2 tablespoons extra-virgin olive oil
½ cups low-sodium chicken broth
½ cup whole pecans
½ cup finely shredded carrot
½ cup finely diced zucchini
1 cup halved cherry tomatoes
¼ cup dried currants

For the vinaigrette:
¼ cup freshly squeezed lemon juice
2 tablespoons minced shallot
Freshly ground black pepper
¾ cup olive or walnut oil

To make the quinoa:

1. Put the quinoa in a fine-mesh sieve, and run cold water over it until the water runs clear. Drain thoroughly and shake out as much water as possible, patting it dry with a paper towel.

2. Heat the olive oil in a large frying pan over medium-high heat. Add the quinoa and toast, stirring frequently, for 2–3 minutes. Be sure to watch closely, as it burns quickly.

3. In a large pot, bring the chicken broth to a boil and add the toasted quinoa. Simmer for 15–17 minutes, adding water to the pot as needed. Drain and transfer to a large bowl.

4. Meanwhile, in a small frying pan over medium-high heat, toast the pecans. Stir frequently to keep them from scorching and remove immediately from the heat once crisp, as they will burn quickly.

5. Add the pecans, carrot, zucchini, tomatoes, and dried currants to the quinoa and mix thoroughly.

To make the vinaigrette:

1. Whisk together the lemon juice and shallots in a small bowl. Add pepper to taste. Drizzle the oil into the mixture in a thin stream, whisking constantly.

2. Pour the vinaigrette over the quinoa and vegetables, and toss thoroughly. Serve immediately.

Pasta Caprese

SERVES 6

▶ *CALORIES PER SERVING* **548** // *SODIUM PER SERVING* **391MG**

This dish is essentially a caprese salad tossed with pasta. The mini mozzarella adds richness, and the tomato and basil bring bright color and nutrients. Use whole-wheat pasta if you're watching your weight and sodium intake. The difference between whole-wheat pasta and white-flour pasta is a whopping 136 milligrams of sodium. The tiny balls of marinated mozzarella used here are called bocconcini, and they also make great appetizers and snacks.

1 pound bocconcini, drained and halved
1 pound small tomatoes, sliced
1 large bunch basil leaves
¾ cup extra-virgin olive oil
Freshly ground black pepper
1 pound whole-wheat spaghetti

1. Put the bocconcini in a large mixing bowl, and add the tomatoes, basil, and olive oil. Toss to combine thoroughly, and season with pepper to taste. Allow the mixture to rest for at least 1 hour to let the cheese soften and flavors develop.

2. Boil the spaghetti according to package instructions and drain. Run cold water over the pasta until the pasta is cool.

3. Add the pasta to the bocconcini mixture along with the basil and toss well.

4. Divide the pasta among 4–6 plates and serve warm or at room temperature.

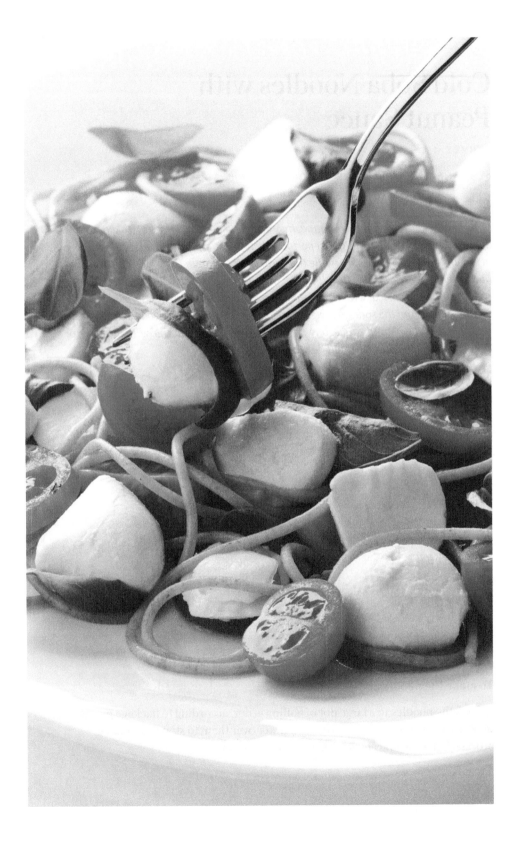

Cold Soba Noodles with Peanut Sauce

SERVES 4

▶ *CALORIES PER SERVING* **476** // *SODIUM PER SERVING* **360MG**

Soba noodles have so much thiamine, they saved the upper classes of Tokyo from dying of beriberi in the Tokugawa period. Their consumption of white rice put them at risk of thiamine deficiency, while the rural poor of Japan thrived because of these buckwheat noodles. To this day, it is a favorite lunch in much of Japan, and it's even catching on in America, with Asian noodle restaurants opening and thriving all over. A word of caution: the sodium levels in soba noodles vary wildly, so be sure to check the label. For the peanut sauce, buy creamy natural peanut butter with no sugar or salt added and the oil separated out.

For the noodles:

1 (8-ounce) package organic soba noodles
Cooking spray
1 red bell pepper, sliced into thin strips
2 cups small broccoli florets
1 cup cilantro leaves
1 small bunch scallions, thinly sliced
1 tablespoon freshly squeezed lime juice, for serving
Chopped unsalted peanuts, for garnish
4 sprigs cilantro, for garnish

For the peanut sauce:

½ cup coconut milk
1 cup creamy natural peanut butter
1 tablespoon freshly squeezed lime juice

To make the noodles:

1. Cook the noodles in a large pot of boiling water, according to package instructions. Drain in a colander and run cold water over them to stop the cooking process. Set aside and cover with a damp dish towel.

2. Spray a large frying pan with cooking spray and place over medium-high heat. When the w is hot, add the bell pepper and sauté until soft, about 5 minutes. Transfer to a bowl and set aside. Spray the pan again and sauté the broccoli just until they are bright green but still firm, 3–5 minutes. Add to the bell pepper.

3. Put the cooled noodles in a large bowl, add the cooked vegetables, and toss well. Stir in the cilantro and scallions.

To make the peanut sauce:

1. Add the coconut milk, peanut butter, and lime juice to a blender or food processor. Process until smooth.

2. Pour the sauce over noodles and toss well to combine. Divide the noodles among 4 bowls, sprinkle a little lime juice over the top, garnish with the peanuts and cilantro sprigs, and serve.

Mini Crab Cakes on Baby Greens

SERVES 6

▸ *CALORIES PER SERVING* **425** // *SODIUM PER SERVING* **248MG**

Crab cakes are a crowd favorite but are often very high in sodium. Here, we bring the crab cakes down to size, decrease the salt, and add red bell pepper, scallions, and parsley to turn them into the perfect hit of protein and vitamin C. Pile two cakes atop a simple green salad rich in iron, vitamin A, and fiber, and lunch is served. Real mayonnaise is called for because the calorie difference between it and light is minimal, but there's more sodium in reduced-fat versions.

For the salad:

1 (5-ounce) package spring greens mix

Extra-virgin olive oil

Balsamic vinegar

Freshly ground black pepper

For the crab cakes:

1 egg, beaten

2–3 tablespoons real mayonnaise

2 green onions, white and green parts finely chopped

1 teaspoon cayenne pepper

3 tablespoons finely chopped red bell pepper

10 butter crackers (such as Ritz or Keebler), finely crushed

¾ pound lump crabmeat

2 tablespoons whole milk

2 tablespoons olive oil

2 tablespoons freshly squeezed lemon juice

2 tablespoons finely chopped parsley leaves

To make the salad:

1. Put the greens in a large bowl and drizzle lightly with olive oil, toss until the leaves are coated. Repeat with the balsamic vinegar, making sure each leaf is lightly dressed. Season with pepper to taste. Divide the salad among 4 plates.

To make the crab cakes:

1. In a large mixing bowl, combine the egg, mayonnaise, green onions, cayenne, bell pepper, and crackers. Mix thoroughly.

2. Break apart and pick through the crabmeat, discarding any shell pieces. Gently fold the milk into the crabmeat. Stir into the egg mixture and incorporate well.

3. Take a heaping tablespoon of crab mixture, pat it into a small patty, and set it on a cutting board or baking sheet. Repeat with the remaining mixture; you should have 8–10 cakes.

4. Heat the oil in a large frying pan over medium-high heat. Add the crab cakes and cook for about 3 minutes on each side. Watch closely and adjust cooking time as needed to avoid burning. Drain the cakes on paper towels.

5. Place 2 warm crab cakes on the center of each plate. Squirt a little lemon on each cake, sprinkle with chopped parsley, and serve immediately.

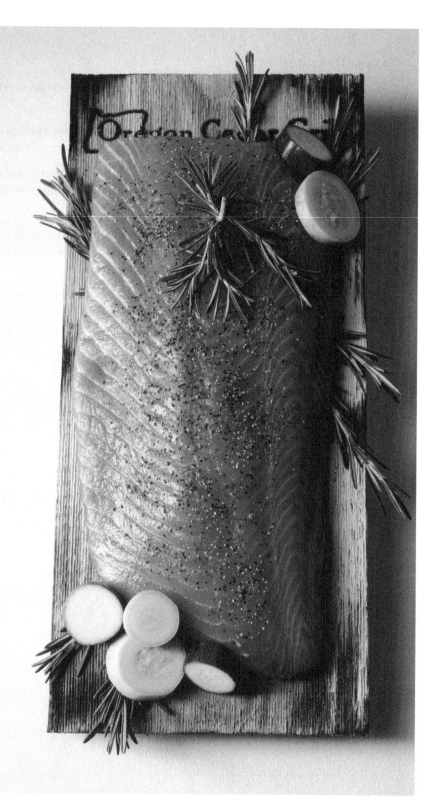

Simple Rosemary Salmon

SERVES 4

▸ *CALORIES PER SERVING* **190** // *SODIUM PER SERVING* **48MG**

The impact of fish on the human body is well documented. Low in calories, it provides large amounts of protein for the body and fatty acids for the brain that boost cognitive function. Buy the freshest fish possible, or if you're landlocked, buy it flash-frozen. In this preparation, the fish is lightly scented with citrus and rosemary and ready to eat in 20 minutes. Serve with a side salad or pan-roasted vegetables for an elegant—and quick—lunch or dinner.

4 (4–5-ounce) salmon fillets
1 orange, very thinly sliced
1 lemon, very thinly sliced
6 sprigs rosemary
1 tablespoon extra-virgin olive oil
Freshly ground black pepper

1. Preheat oven to 400 degrees F.

2. Rinse the salmon under cold running water and pat dry with paper towels.

3. In the bottom of a shallow baking dish, make an alternating layer of lemon and orange slices. Lay the rosemary sprigs evenly on top and arrange the salmon fillets over them. Drizzle each fillet with a little olive oil, and season with black pepper to taste.

4. Bake for 20 minutes, or until the salmon flakes easily with a fork. Place 1 fillet on each of 4 plates. Drizzle any pan juices over the salmon, if desired. Serve immediately.

Noodle Salad with Shrimp and Cucumber

SERVES 4

▶ *CALORIES PER SERVING* **280** // *SODIUM PER SERVING* **298MG**

In this recipe, shrimp is gently boiled in spiced oil and vinegar and then paired with cool cucumber. Always in cooking, think opposites—spicy and mild, sweet and sour, smooth and crunchy—to create interesting, sensual food.

2 cups whole-wheat pasta, such as penne or fusilli

¼ cup white wine vinegar

2 garlic cloves, finely chopped

2 tablespoons dried oregano

¼ cup extra-virgin olive oil

1 pound shrimp, peeled and deveined

1 cucumber, peeled, seeded, quartered lengthwise, and thinly sliced

1. In a large pot of boiling water, cook the pasta until al dente according to the package directions. Do not overcook. Drain and run cold water over the pasta to stop the cooking. Drain again, and then transfer to a large bowl.

2. In a small bowl, stir together the vinegar, garlic, and oregano. Slowly drizzle in the oil, whisking constantly. Pour into a small skillet and place over medium heat. Add the shrimp to the hot oil mixture and cook until they turn pink, about 3 minutes.

3. Add the shrimp, along with the oil mixture, to the pasta, stir in the cucumber, and toss the salad thoroughly to coat. Serve at room temperature or chill for 30 to 60 minutes before serving.

Spicy Chickpeas and Turkey

SERVES 4

▸ *CALORIES PER SERVING* **530** // *SODIUM PER SERVING* **389MG**

Chickpeas are nutty, toothsome legumes grown primarily in India, Pakistan, and Turkey. They are a cornerstone of the Middle Eastern diet in the form of falafel, among many other things. They are also powerful protein providers, making them an excellent entrée. Chickpeas are perfect paired with sausages, but here, lean ground turkey keeps the sodium levels down and makes this dish a light and delightful lunch. Note that you need to plan ahead when making this recipe, as the chickpeas must soak overnight.

1 pound dried chickpeas

2 tablespoons extra-virgin olive oil

1 large yellow onion, chopped

1 clove garlic, minced

1 pound lean ground turkey

½ cup red wine

1 (28-ounce) can whole tomatoes

1 teaspoon fresh thyme leaves

2 tablespoons red pepper flakes

Freshly ground black pepper

Freshly squeezed lemon juice (optional)

4 thyme sprigs, for garnish

1. The night before making the soup, put the chickpeas in a large pot or bowl and cover with water. Let them soak overnight. Drain and set aside.

2. Heat the olive oil in a large Dutch oven over medium-high heat. When very hot, add the onion and garlic and cook until soft and translucent, about 5 minutes.

3. Crumble the ground turkey into the pan and cook until just brown. Remove the pan from the heat.

4. Add the red wine, tomatoes, thyme, red pepper flakes, and black pepper to taste, and stir well to incorporate. Return the pan to the heat and cook for 5 minutes at a low simmer, stirring frequently.

continued ▸

5. Add the chickpeas, return to a simmer, cover, and cook for 30–40 minutes. Check the chickpeas for doneness: they should be easy to chew but still firm. Squeeze fresh lemon juice over the top, if desired.

6. Serve immediately in large shallow bowls, and garnish with the thyme sprigs. This dish is also great after a night in the refrigerator; reheat before serving.

Turkey Burgers with Cranberry-Scallion Sauce

SERVES 4

▸ *CALORIES PER SERVING* **472** // *SODIUM PER SERVING* **307MG**

Dry, overcooked turkey has given turkey burgers a bad name. Here, the dry factor has been overcome by adding egg whites that give the patties texture, more protein, and plumpness. Still, when making this recipe, keep an eye on the burgers while cooking and be sure to remove them from the pan as soon as they're done. If your tastes are strictly savory, you can forgo the sweet sauce; instead, top the burgers with fat slices of red onion and tomato and experiment with flavored mayonnaise.

For the burgers:

2 pounds lean ground turkey

2 egg whites, lightly beaten

¼ cup diced onion

½ cup chopped parsley leaves

½ teaspoon cayenne pepper

Freshly ground black pepper

Cooking spray

4 whole-wheat English muffins, split and toasted

For the sauce:

1 cup whole-berry cranberry sauce

1 tablespoon finely grated orange zest

2 scallions, chopped

To make the burgers:

1. Put the ground turkey in a large bowl and add the egg whites. Using clean hands, knead the egg whites into the turkey. Add the onion, parsley, and cayenne. Season with black pepper to taste and continue kneading until well incorporated. Divide the mixture into 4 equal parts and form into patties about 1 inch thick.

continued ▶

2. Spray a large frying pan with cooking spray and place over medium-high heat. Cook the burgers for 6–7 minutes on each side, or until the meat is no longer pink. Drain on paper towels.

To make the sauce:

1. In a small bowl, whisk together the cranberry sauce, orange zest, and scallions. Set aside.

2. To assemble, put a burger on half of an English muffin, spoon sauce onto the patty, top with the other muffin half, and serve

Lightning-Fast Chicken Stir-Fry

SERVES 6

▶ *CALORIES PER SERVING* **111** *(***327** *WITH BROWN RICE)*
▶ *SODIUM PER SERVING* **382MG** *(***392MG** *WITH BROWN RICE)*

After you've prepared this recipe once or twice, it becomes so simple you could do it in your sleep. The vegetables in this recipe can be any combination you choose: bell peppers, pea shoots, cauliflower, zucchini, asparagus, peas, corn, tomatoes, and so on. The brown rice is not crucial and totally optional—the stir-fry is great with or without it. A word of caution: the sodium levels in low-sodium chicken broth vary wildly, so be sure to check the label.

1 (14.5-ounce) can low-sodium chicken broth
¼ cup low-sodium soy sauce
2 garlic cloves, smashed
2 tablespoons cornstarch
1 teaspoon ground ginger
¼ teaspoon ground nutmeg
1 tablespoon peanut oil
1½ pounds skinless, boneless chicken breast, cut into thin strips
4 cups coarsely chopped broccoli or mixed vegetables
2 cups cooked brown rice (optional)

1. In a medium bowl, whisk together the chicken broth, soy sauce, garlic, cornstarch, ginger, and nutmeg until smooth.

2. Heat the oil in a large skillet or wok over medium-high heat. When the oil is hot, add the chicken and cook, stirring frequently, until cooked through, about 3 minutes. Stir-fry in batches if needed. Add the broccoli to the pan and cook, stirring frequently, for 5 minutes.

3. Pour the chicken broth mixture over the chicken and vegetables and increase the heat to high. Let the sauce boil rapidly for about 1 minute. Remove the pan from the heat and serve the stir-fry with brown rice, if desired.

Chicken Curry

SERVES 4

▸ *CALORIES PER SERVING* **299** // *SODIUM PER SERVING* **44MG**

A "true" curry is about a balance rather than the overwhelming power of one spice. It also becomes more delicious with time. Flavors meld and deepen. Make this dish the night before, and let sit in the refrigerator overnight. Reheat and serve with hot brown rice. Have small bowls with the garnishes ready to sprinkle over the curry, if desired. Garam masala is an Indian spice mixture available in large grocery stores and gourmet markets.

2 tablespoons peanut oil

1 large onion, thinly sliced

1 cup tomatoes, chopped

1 tablespoon minced fresh garlic

1 tablespoon peeled, finely diced fresh ginger

2 teaspoons garam masala

1 teaspoon ground turmeric

3–3½ pounds boneless, skinless chicken breasts, cut into bite-sized pieces

½ cup low-fat plain yogurt

1 cup water

1–2 teaspoons red pepper flakes

4 cups cooked long-grain brown rice

Hard-boiled eggs, chopped

Peanuts or cashews, chopped

Red onion, diced

Cilantro leaves, chopped

Parsley leaves, chopped

Shredded coconut

Chutney

1. Heat the peanut oil in a large frying pan over medium-high heat.

2. As the pan gets hot, separate the onion rings and add them to the pan. Cook for 7–10 minutes, or until golden brown.

continued ▸

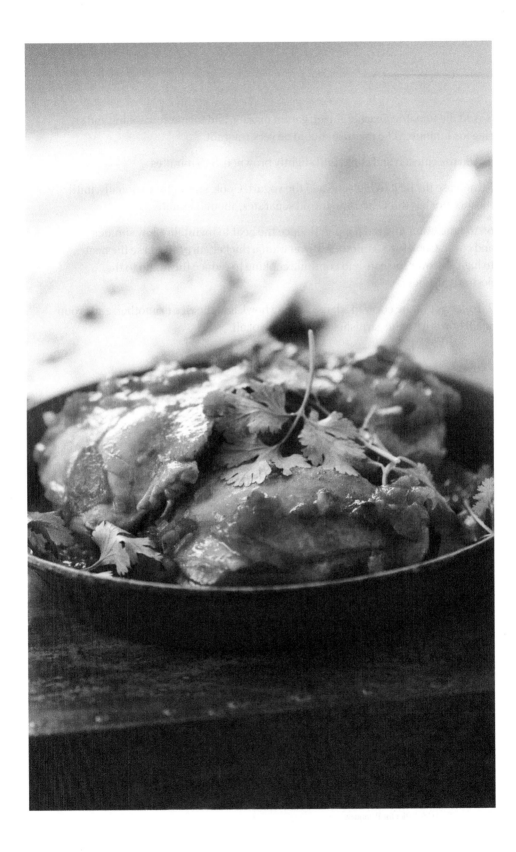

3. Add the tomatoes, garlic, ginger, garam masala, and turmeric, cooking and stirring for 1 minute. The mixture should be very fragrant.

4. Add the chicken and cook until slightly browned, 3–5 minutes.

5. Increase the heat to high and add the yogurt. Cook, stirring occasionally, until the mixture has thickened and the oil separates, about 5 minutes.

6. Add the water and red pepper. Reduce the heat to maintain a low simmer and cover. Cook for 30 minutes. If you want a thicker curry, increase the heat to high, uncover the pan, and continue cooking to reduce the liquid to the desired thickness.

7. To serve, put the curry in a large serving bowl, and the rice in another, and group small bowls with the garnishes within reach of all.

Vietnamese Pork Sandwiches

SERVES 4

▸ *CALORIES PER SERVING* **339** // *SODIUM PER SERVING* **474MG**

Pork tenderloin is a perfect cut of meat for the busy individual. It cooks in about 20 minutes in the oven or on the grill and is equally suitable as the centerpiece of a meal or sliced and tucked into wraps or salads. Fresh vegetables add crunch, fiber, and nutrients—as well as a Vietnamese touch—to this sandwich. This is usually piled on a French baguette, but use a whole-wheat version here to bring down the excessive sodium content of commercially baked white bread.

1–1½ pounds boneless pork tenderloin

Extra-virgin olive oil, for coating

2 (18-inch) whole-wheat baguettes or 4 whole-wheat sandwich buns

2¼ cup real mayonnaise

1 teaspoon low-sodium chili sauce

¼ cup freshly squeezed lime juice

1 red onion, thinly sliced

1 large cucumber, peeled, halved lengthwise, seeds removed, and thinly sliced

2 tablespoons fresh cilantro leaves

Freshly ground black pepper

1. Preheat oven to 425 degrees F.

2. Coat all sides of the tenderloin with the olive oil, place in a baking dish, and roast for 15–20 minutes. Watch it closely for doneness: tenderloins dry out fast. Let rest for 5 minutes and then slice thinly.

3. Cut the baguettes into 9-inch-long sections and halve lengthwise.

4. Spread the mayonnaise on both insides of the baguette sections. Place 2–3 pork slices on one side, and spread a quarter of the chili sauce over the pork. Drizzle with a little lime juice. Layer a quarter of the onion, cucumber, and fresh cilantro leaves, and season with pepper to taste. Finish with another drizzle of lime juice. Repeat for the remaining sandwiches. Serve immediately.

Soft Beef Tacos

SERVES 4

▶ *CALORIES PER SERVING* **632** // *SODIUM PER SERVING* **161MG**

In Mexico, the days are hot and the tacos are made with soft tortillas, not commercially processed crispy corn shells from a box. The perfect delivery device for lean meats, vegetables, herbs, and cheeses, the humble corn tortilla should be celebrated and enjoyed.

1½–2 pounds flank steak
1 cup freshly squeezed lime juice
2 tablespoons ground cumin
2 tablespoons ground coriander
2 tablespoons ground black pepper
4 ears corn, shucked
1 tomato, chopped
8 corn tortillas
1 cup cilantro leaves
1 cup diced red onion
1 medium avocado, pitted and diced
Hot sauce (optional)

1. The day before making the tacos, put the steak in a large sealable plastic bag. Add the lime juice and let stand in the refrigerator overnight. The acid will break down this tougher cut of meat and gently flavor it.

2. Preheat broiler or grill for 10 minutes.

3. Drain the lime juice and pat the flank steak dry with paper towels.

4. In a small bowl, combine the cumin, coriander, and pepper. Rub the mixture all over the steak.

5. Broil or grill the steak for 13–18 minutes, depending on whether you want it cooked rare or medium well. Transfer to a plate and let rest for 10 minutes.

6. Meanwhile, set the base of a corn cob in a large, deep bowl, holding the corn upright. With a sharp knife, slice the kernels off the cob. Repeat with the remaining corn cobs, catching the juices in the bowl.

7. Add the tomato to the corn. Mix gently and set aside to let the flavors blend.

8. Cut the steak in thin slices on an extreme diagonal. Place a few steak strips on a tortilla, and top with 1 tablespoon each of the corn-tomato mixture, cilantro, onion, and avocado. Repeat with the remaining tortillas. Serve immediately, passing the hot sauce, if desired.

Bobotie Lite

SERVES 4 TO 6

▶ *CALORIES PER SERVING* **557** // *SODIUM PER SERVING* **253MG**

Bobotie is a much-beloved spiced meat casserole throughout Africa. The ingredients here are lighter than the traditional regional versions, with low-sodium substitutes, but the dish is plenty hearty and satisfying, regardless of where you live. Serve the Bobotie with rice and garnish with fresh coconut, chutney, and cashews.

2 tablespoons margarine

2 large onions, chopped

1 slice ciabatta bread

1 cup fat-free milk, divided

2 pounds ground beef

⅓ cup seedless raisins

¼ cup dried apricots

¼ cup coarsely chopped almonds

¼ cup freshly squeezed lemon juice

2 tablespoons curry powder

2 large eggs

1. Preheat the oven to 350° F.

2. Melt the margarine in a large skillet over medium heat. Add the onions and cook until soft and translucent.

3. Meanwhile, in a large bowl, soak the ciabatta in ½ cup of the milk.

4. Transfer the cooked onions to the bowl with the bread. Add the beef, raisins, apricots, almonds, lemon juice, and curry powder and mix thoroughly to combine. Transfer the mixture to a 9 × 13-inch casserole dish.

5. Beat the eggs with the remaining ½ cup of milk and pour over the casserole. Bake for 45 minutes. Let sit for 5 minutes before serving.

Filet Mignon with Red Wine au Jus

SERVES 4

▶ *CALORIES PER SERVING* **299** // *SODIUM PER SERVING* **328MG**

Save this recipe for when the mother-in-law or boss comes for lunch. This cut of beef is expensive and extra lean. It overcooks quickly; even fifteen seconds too long on the heat can dry it out, so vigilance and speed are essential. This recipe also explains the basic technique for creating au jus sauce. Use it over and over on any cut of meat, poultry, or game. Since filets have so little fat, a sauce is often spooned over the top to add moisture and flavor. Add some sautéed asparagus or steamed haricots verts and you have one sophisticated lunch.

4 (3-ounce) filets mignons
Cooking spray
1–2 tablespoons extra-virgin olive oil
¼ cup chopped shallots
1 cup low-sodium beef broth
½ cup red wine

1. Spray both sides of the steaks with a thin sheen of cooking spray. Let them sit at room temperature for 30–60 minutes.

2. Heat a large frying pan over medium-high heat until very hot. Add the filets and sear on one side for about 1 minute. Flip and sear the other side. Reduce the heat to medium and cook the steaks, uncovered, for 10–13 minutes. Watch them very carefully. Filets are usually cooked medium-rare for maximum juiciness, but they are also delicious cooked medium or medium-well. Transfer the steaks to 4 plates, reserving the pan drippings.

continued ▶

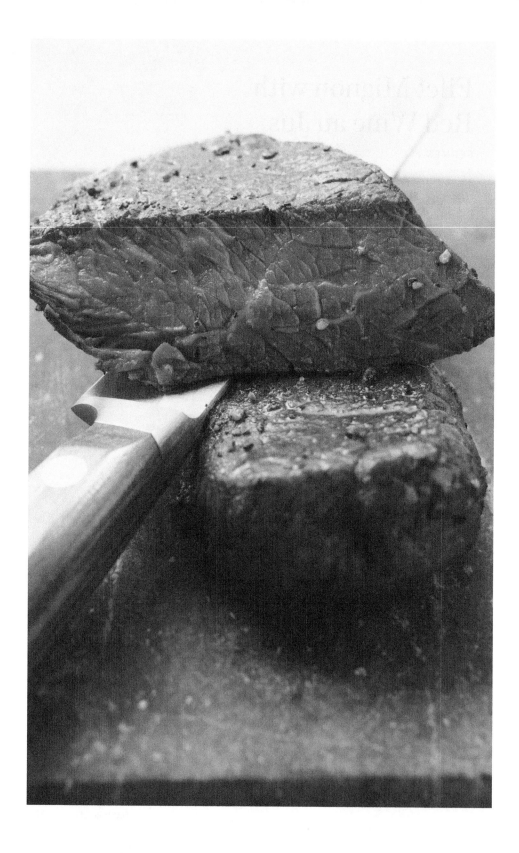

3. Working quickly, return the steak pan with drippings to medium-high heat and add the olive oil and shallots. Cook the shallots until soft and translucent, 2–3 minutes. Slowly add in the beef broth and wine, stirring to combine. Scrape the bottom and sides of the pan with a spoon to release any brown bits. Reduce the heat to low and simmer until the pan sauce thickens enough to coat the back of a spoon.

4. Pour the sauce over the filets and serve immediately.

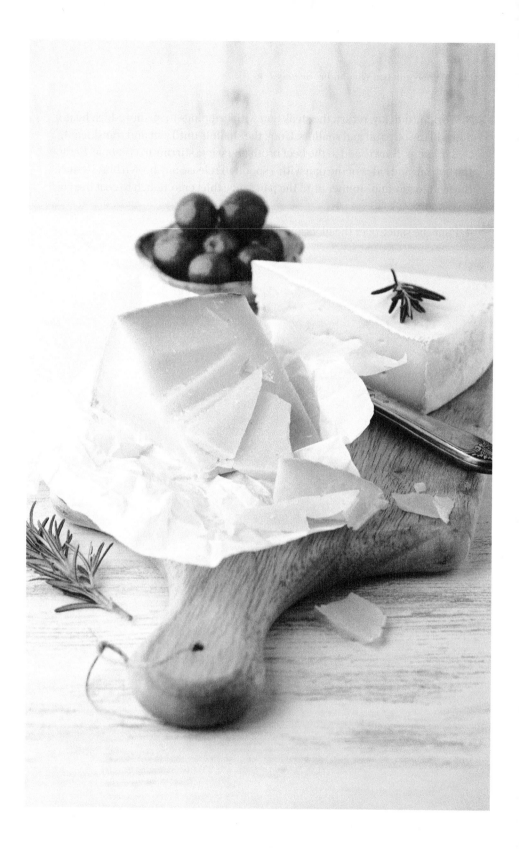

CHAPTER FOURTEEN

DASH Snacks and Appetizers

- Agua Fresca
- Red, White, and Blue Fruit Kebabs
- Spice-Roasted Sunflower and Pumpkin Seeds
- Spiced Edamame
- Sweet-Hot Maple Almonds
- Cajun Popcorn
- Vegetable Smoothie
- Cucumber Gazpacho
- Pickled Cucumbers
- Vegetable Chips
- Baked Chili-Lime Tortilla Chips
- Baked Applesauce with Walnuts
- Strawberry-Mango Salsa with Basil
- Watermelon and Pistachio Salad
- Tomato Salsa with Jalapeños and Lime

- Onion and Herb Dip
- Roasted Red Pepper Dip
- Spicy Oil-Roasted Chickpeas
- Homemade Hummus with Crudités
- Herbed Deviled Eggs
- Watercress Tea Sandwiches with Sweet-Hot Mayonnaise
- Cilantro-Avocado Tea Sandwiches
- Simple Lobster Tea Sandwiches
- Cucumber and Dill Tea Sandwiches
- Shrimp and Mango "Ceviche"
- Turkey Mozzarella Shooters
- Tiny Turkey Quesadillas
- Lemon-Glazed Tiny Drumsticks
- Thai Pork in Lettuce Wraps
- DASH Meatballs

Agua Fresca

SERVES 4

▶ *CALORIES PER SERVING* **283** // *SODIUM PER SERVING* **26MG**

Turn to restorative drinks when you need an afternoon pick-me-up that will take you through to dinnertime. In Mexico, chunks of fresh fruit are whirled together and sold as agua fresca, which means "cooling water." Try replacing the watermelon with mango, papaya, or pineapple. You can also pack in extra nutrition by adding chia seeds.

8 cups chopped seedless watermelon, chilled
1 cup cranberry nectar
¼ cup freshly squeezed lime juice
1 or 2 ice cubes (optional)
Mint leaves (optional)

1. Place the watermelon, cranberry nectar, and lime juice in a blender, and blend until smooth. Add the ice cubes if needed, but if the watermelon is cold enough, they won't be necessary. Strain the mixture through a fine-mesh sieve into glasses. Garnish with mint leaves, if desired, and serve immediately.

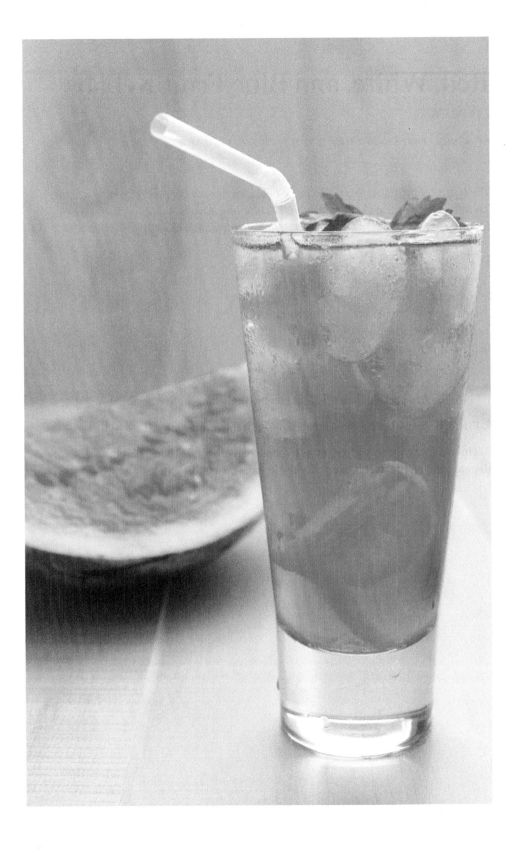

Red, White, and Blue Fruit Kebabs

SERVES 4

▶ *CALORIES PER SERVING* **176** // *SODIUM PER SERVING* **4MG**

The beauty of this snack lies in the ingredients: use the very best of the season's fruits. These kebabs will give delight through the color and flavor combinations you create. Use long wooden skewers for the kebabs; they are available at most grocery stores.

1 pint strawberries, hulled
2 tablespoons balsamic vinegar
2 bananas, peeled and cut into 2-inch pieces
Juice of 1 small orange
1 pint blueberries

1. Place the strawberries in a medium bowl with the balsamic vinegar. Toss well.

2. Place the banana pieces in a small bowl with the orange juice. Toss well.

3. Thread a strawberry onto a skewer, then a banana piece, then a blueberry. Repeat until all the fruit is used. Lay the kebabs on a platter and serve.

Spice-Roasted Sunflower and Pumpkin Seeds

SERVES 4

▶ *CALORIES PER SERVING* **480** // *SODIUM PER SERVING* **176MG**

In some other cultures, as well as most baseball dugouts, sunflower seed shells litter the ground, but despite their many health benefits, seeds have not made it into the American diet in a significant way yet. Try this recipe: it may change your mind. Sprinkle these spiced seeds on salads and in soups.

¼ cup extra-virgin olive oil

1 tablespoon tamari

1 tablespoon chili powder

2 teaspoons garlic powder

1 teaspoon cayenne pepper

Zest of 1 lime

2 cups raw sunflower seeds

1 cup raw pumpkin seeds

1. Preheat the oven to 350° F.

2. In a small bowl, whisk together the oil, tamari, chili powder, garlic powder, cayenne, and lime zest. Pour the mixture into a sealable plastic bag. Add the sunflower and pumpkin seeds, seal the top, and shake and turn the bag until the seeds are well coated.

3. Spread the seeds in a single layer on a rimmed baking sheet or in a shallow roasting pan. Roast for 15 minutes, stirring once halfway through. Check the seeds often during roasting so they don't burn.

4. Let the seeds cool to room temperature. They can be stored in an airtight container for up to 1 week.

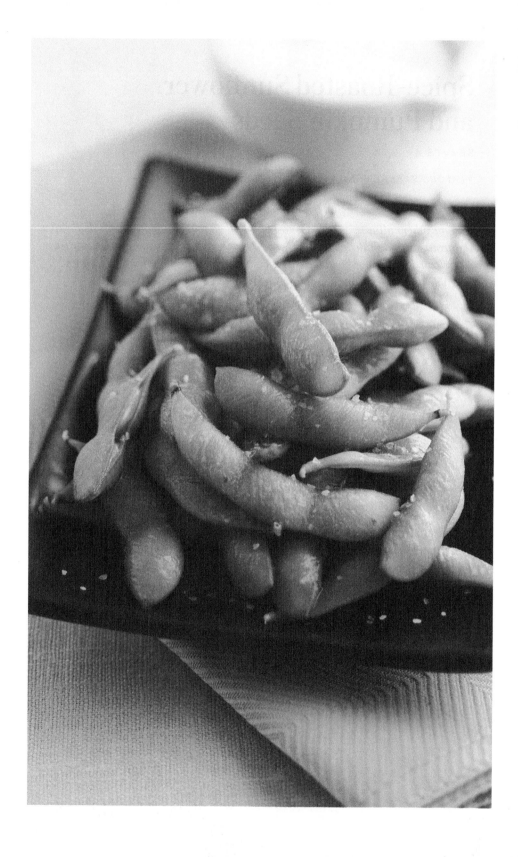

Spiced Edamame

SERVES 4

▶ *CALORIES PER SERVING* **243** // *SODIUM PER SERVING* **250MG**

Edamame is the immature soybean in the pod, and it is featured in the cuisines of Japan, China, and Hawaii. You can cook and season the pods, as we do here, for snacking, or cook the shelled soybeans to use in salads and side dishes. To eat them from the pod, simply bite down on one end and pull the pod out between your clenched teeth. The beans pop out into your mouth along with the gentle flavors from the cooking broth.

3 garlic cloves, coarsely chopped

2 tablespoons low-sodium soy sauce

2 tablespoons unseasoned rice vinegar

1 tablespoon brown sugar

1 (10- to 14-ounce) package frozen edamame, thawed

1 tablespoon chili powder

1 teaspoon crushed red pepper flakes

½ teaspoon dried oregano

1. Fill a medium pot half full with water and bring to a boil over medium-high heat. Add the garlic, soy sauce, rice vinegar, and brown sugar and stir well. Add the edamame and boil for 6–8 minutes, or until firm-tender. Drain well.

2. Transfer the edamame to a medium bowl and sprinkle with the chili powder, red pepper flakes, and oregano. Toss well to coat the pods evenly with the spices. Serve immediately.

Sweet-Hot Maple Almonds

SERVES 6

▶ *CALORIES PER SERVING* **521** // *SODIUM PER SERVING* **289MG**

Almonds are a perfect snack food when you're on a healthy diet. In this recipe, the renowned Asian flavor combination of sweet-hot—accomplished here by combining soy sauce and maple syrup—bakes into the nuts and turns them a deep mahogany color.

1 pound raw almonds
5 tablespoons maple syrup
2 tablespoons reduced-sodium soy sauce
1 teaspoon cayenne pepper
Cooking spray

1. Preheat the oven to 350° F.

2. Spread the almonds in a single layer on a rimmed baking sheet and bake for 6–7 minutes. Let the almonds cool slightly.

3. In a large bowl, whisk together the maple syrup, soy sauce, and cayenne. Add the almonds to the bowl and stir well until thoroughly coated.

4. Thinly coat the baking sheet with cooking spray. Spread the almonds in the pan in a single layer and roast for 15–17 minutes, stirring every few minutes, until the nuts turn a deep brown. Let the almonds cool to room temperature and serve in small bowls.

Cajun Popcorn

SERVES 8

▶ *CALORIES PER SERVING* **137** // *SODIUM PER SERVING* **44MG**

This popcorn is flavored with intense spices and is a perfect pairing with ice-cold beer or lemonade. Serve it in small amounts—the taste is strong and satisfying. Popcorn is in the mix at the hip bars of New York City, but somehow it always tastes better at home. The calorie count is based on popcorn popped in canola oil. Air popping brings each cup down a full 20 calories. The choice is yours.

2 tablespoons extra-virgin olive oil
2 tablespoons margarine
1 teaspoon paprika
1 teaspoon lemon pepper
½ to 1 teaspoon cayenne pepper
1 teaspoon ground cumin
10 cups popped corn

1. In a small saucepan, heat the olive oil and margarine over medium heat until melted. Add the paprika, lemon pepper, cayenne, and cumin, and mix thoroughly. Reduce the heat to low and let the spices steep for about 5 minutes.

2. Pour the spiced oil over the popcorn, toss well with your hands or salad spoons to coat, and divide among bowls to serve.

Vegetable Smoothie

SERVES 2

▶ *CALORIES PER SERVING* **273** // *SODIUM PER SERVING* **196MG**

Sweet smoothies may be what you prefer in the morning, but a savory smoothie or power-packed vegetable juice blend are just the thing for sustained energy through the long afternoon. If you want yours to be more smoothie than juice, use ice cubes instead of cold water. Wash all the produce thoroughly under running water to get rid of any contaminants. Better still, use all organic.

4 or 5 cherry tomatoes
½ bunch parsley with stems
2 to 3 large handfuls spinach leaves
1 stalk celery, coarsely chopped
½ jalapeño pepper, seeded (optional)
½ avocado
Juice of 1 lemon
Cold water
½ cup low-fat plain yogurt

1. In a blender, combine the tomatoes, parsley, spinach, celery, jalapeño, avocado, and lemon juice, and blend for 2 minutes, or until smooth. Add cold water a little at a time until the smoothie reaches the desired consistency. Add the yogurt, pulse briefly to incorporate, and serve.

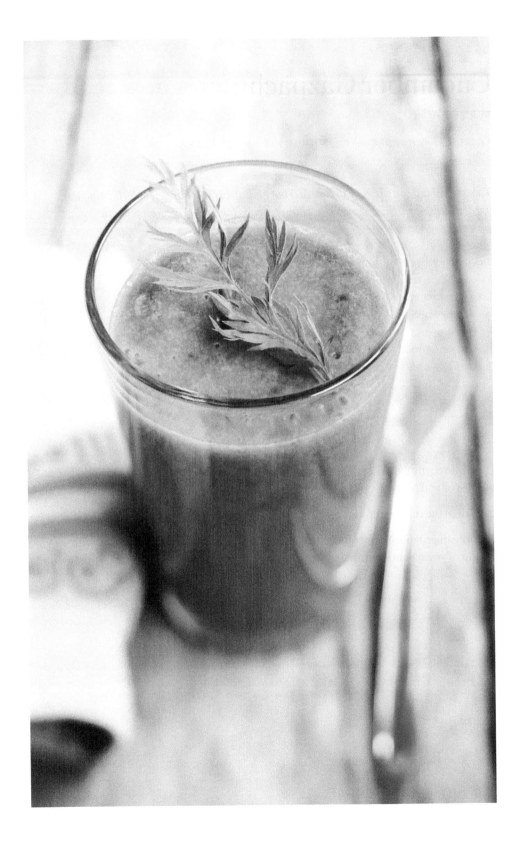

Cucumber Gazpacho

SERVES 4

▶ *CALORIES PER SERVING 78 // SODIUM PER SERVING 56MG*

This refreshing soup is easy to love in a hot climate. If you happen to be hosting the garden club, serve the gazpacho in china teacups for a most elegant pick-me-up.

3 cups chopped English cucumber
2 cups grape tomatoes
1 cup fat-free, low-sodium chicken broth
¼ cup chopped onion
1 garlic clove, chopped
¼ teaspoon ground cumin
¼ teaspoon paprika
Ground white pepper
1 cup whole-milk plain yogurt, for garnish
¼ cup chopped fresh cilantro leaves, for garnish

1. Put the cucumber, tomatoes, broth, onion, garlic, cumin, and paprika in a food processor and process until smooth.

2. Cool in the refrigerator for at least 2 hours and preferably 6 hours before serving.

3. Ladle the gazpacho into chilled bowls, season with white pepper, garnish with a dollop of yogurt and a sprinkle of cilantro, and serve.

Pickled Cucumbers

SERVES 4

▶ *CALORIES PER SERVING* **69** // *SODIUM PER SERVING* **0MG**

This is a good basic recipe for any firm vegetable that can be marinated and tucked into a sandwich, thrown in a salad, or piled on a crudités platter. Here we use the traditional cucumbers, but jicama, cauliflower florets, and carrot coins are delicious alternatives. Try adding chopped herbs for additional flavor. Store them in a large mason jar (fully submerged in the vinegar mixture) in the refrigerator for about 1 week.

½ cup unseasoned rice vinegar
¼ cup sugar
2 English cucumbers, peeled and sliced into 1-inch-thick coins

1. Put the vinegar in a small saucepan over medium heat and bring to a boil. Stir in the sugar and boil until it is completely dissolved.

2. Put the cucumber coins in a medium bowl. Pour the vinegar marinade over the top. If the liquid does not cover all the pieces, be sure to stir the contents every few hours. Cover and marinate the cucumbers in the refrigerator overnight. Serve.

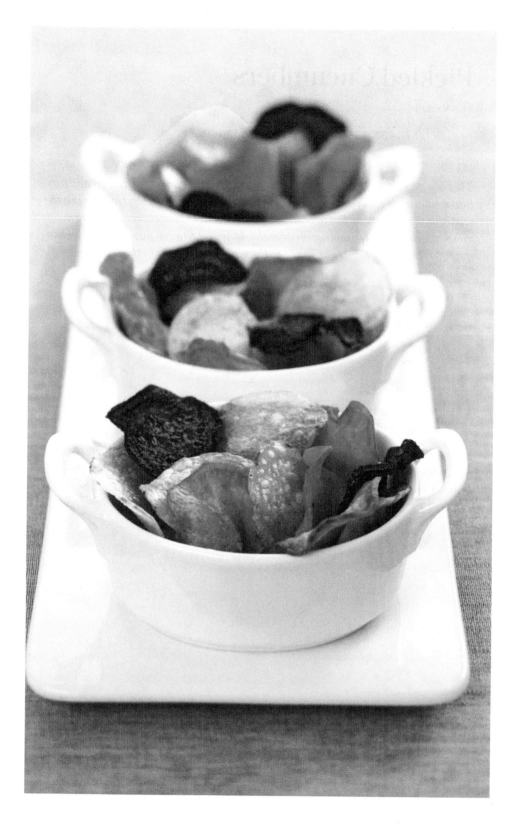

Vegetable Chips

SERVES 8

▶ *CALORIES PER SERVING* **205** // *SODIUM PER SERVING* **143MG**

To make these chips, vegetables are sliced razor thin (a mandoline or really sharp knife helps) and slowly dried out in the oven until crispy. Use sturdier vegetables, such as zucchini and sweet potatoes, if serving the chips with a dip. Wash the vegetables thoroughly and do not peel them (except for the beets); the skin provides even more nutrients and fiber. Select any combination of your favorite vegetables for drying. The calorie and sodium estimates are based on a ½-cup serving.

2 cups thinly sliced zucchini or other squash
2 cups thinly sliced sweet potatoes
2 cups thinly sliced turnips
2 cups peeled, thinly sliced beets
2 cups kale leaves or collard greens, ribs removed and torn into bite-sized pieces
About ¼ cup extra-virgin olive oil

1. Preheat the oven to 275° F.

2. To prepare the zucchini, sweet potatoes, turnips, and beets for baking, first spread the vegetables on paper towels, salt well (it's rinsed off later), and let sit for at least 30 minutes. The salt draws moisture out of the vegetables, which helps them to crisp up.

3. Rinse the vegetables under cold running water to remove the salt, and then dry them completely on paper towels. The drier the vegetables, the better the results.

4. To prepare the greens, rinse them in a colander under cold running water and spread them on paper towels to dry completely. Drying them well makes the crispest chips.

5. Spread the vegetables in a single layer on a rimmed baking sheet (bake in batches as needed) and drizzle with the olive oil, coating each piece. Bake for 1 hour, turning the vegetables once halfway through the cooking. Transfer to paper towels to drain and cool. Serve within 2 hours, or store in an airtight container for 1–2 days.

Baked Chili-Lime Tortilla Chips

SERVES 4

▶ *CALORIES PER SERVING* **168** // *SODIUM PER SERVING* **134MG**

Given a choice between French fries and tortilla chips, many Americans would be hard pressed to pick a favorite. Luckily, we can take deep-fried out of the equation to comply with DASH and create these delicious chips—full of flavor for snacking on by themselves or equally perfect for scooping up a dip or salsa.

12 (6-inch) corn tortillas
3 tablespoons canola or other vegetable oil
1 tablespoon chili powder
1 tablespoon lime zest
1 teaspoon cayenne pepper

1. Preheat the oven to 350° F.

2. Cut each tortilla into 6 wedges using kitchen shears or a sharp knife.

3. In a medium bowl, whisk together the oil, chili powder, lime zest, and cayenne. Dip the tortilla wedges in the oil mixture and spread in a single layer on 2 baking sheets or shallow roasting pans.

4. Bake for 20–25 minutes, or until the chips are browned and crunchy. Transfer to paper towels to drain and cool before serving.

Baked Applesauce with Walnuts

SERVES 6

▶ *CALORIES PER SERVING* **386** // *SODIUM PER SERVING* **0MG**

There are many different ways to make applesauce, but if the apples are baked rather than boiled, it gives the applesauce a flavor like that of an apple pie or crumble. Try several varieties of apples to change the flavor nuances and discover your personal favorite.

Cooking spray
3 pounds apples, halved and cored
2 tablespoons brown sugar
1 to 2 teaspoons ground cinnamon
Juice of ½ lemon
½ cup walnut pieces, for garnish

1. Preheat the oven to 375° F.

2. Thinly coat a rimmed baking sheet with cooking spray. Place the apples cut side down on the pan and bake for 30 minutes. Let cool slightly.

3. When the apples are cool enough to handle, pick them up by the softened skins and squeeze the apple flesh onto the cookie sheet. Discard the skins.

4. Transfer the apples to a large bowl and add the brown sugar, cinnamon, and lemon juice. Mash the mixture with a fork to combine. If you prefer perfectly smooth applesauce, process in batches in a food processor.

5. To serve, dish the applesauce into small bowls or cups and garnish with the walnuts.

Strawberry-Mango Salsa with Basil

SERVES 4

▶ *CALORIES PER SERVING* **46** *// SODIUM PER SERVING* **1MG**

A perfect counterpoint to spicy tomato salsa, this fruity version can also be on the table and your guests will enjoy the differences between them. The play of spicy versus sweet can be a powerful combination.

1 cup chopped strawberries
1 cup chopped mango
1 jalapeño pepper, finely diced
¼ cup finely chopped red onion
¼ cup shredded basil leaves
2 tablespoons freshly squeezed lemon juice
Freshly ground pepper

1. Combine all of the ingredients in a medium bowl and mix thoroughly. Cover and refrigerate for 2–4 hours to let the flavors blend before serving.

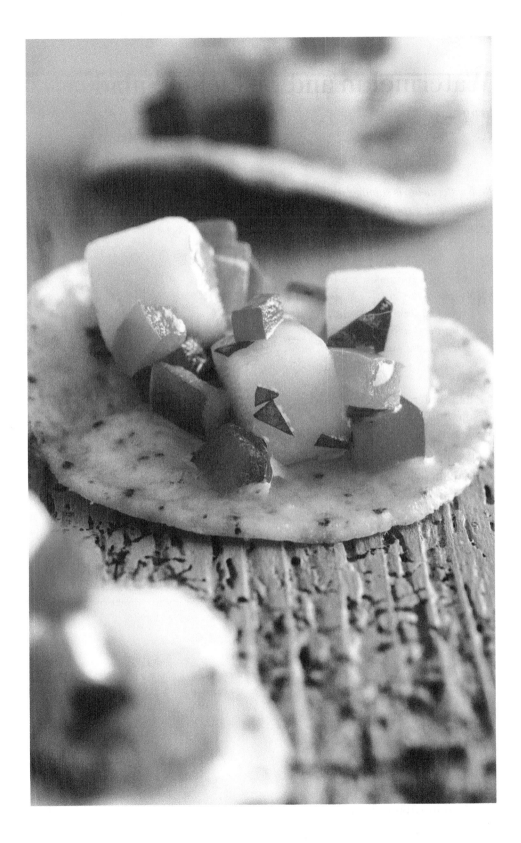

Watermelon and Pistachio Salad

SERVES 4

▶ *CALORIES PER SERVING* **285** // *SODIUM PER SERVING* **130MG**

Ripe watermelon is summer itself. Sweet and juicy, watermelon responds well to the crunch of a dry-roasted pistachio. Cut the watermelon chunks larger than you would for a fruit salad—this is finger food.

10 cups ripe watermelon, cut in 2 x 2-inch chunks
1 tablespoon lime zest
2 tablespoons lime juice
Freshly ground pepper
1 cup dry-roasted, unsalted pistachios

1. Put the watermelon chunks in a large bowl. Add the lime zest and juice and season with pepper. Stir gently with a large spatula to coat the watermelon without breaking them.

2. Place the pistachio nuts in a sealable plastic bag or wrap them in a kitchen towel. Run a rolling pin over them to break them up, keeping the pieces as big as possible. Sprinkle the pistachios over the watermelon and serve immediately.

Tomato Salsa with Jalapeños and Lime

SERVES 4

▶ *CALORIES PER SERVING* **123** // *SODIUM PER SERVING* **10MG**

Simple, nutritious, and packed with flavor, salsa is destined for marriage to a baked tortilla chip. Try thinking outside the box. Stir it into mayonnaise for a sandwich spread, spoon it over burgers, or toss it in a salad as dressing.

¼ cup chopped onions

2 garlic cloves, finely chopped

4 large ripe tomatoes, peeled, seeded, and chopped

1-4 jalapeño peppers, seeded and finely diced

¼ cup chopped cilantro leaves

2 tablespoons freshly squeezed lime juice

1 tablespoon extra-virgin olive oil

1 tablespoon white vinegar

1 teaspoon ground cumin

1. Place the onions and garlic in a colander and pour 2 cups boiling water over them. Drain well and transfer to a large bowl.

2. Add the tomatoes, jalapeños, cilantro, lime juice, olive oil, vinegar, and cumin, and mix thoroughly. Cover and refrigerate for 2–4 hours to let the flavors blend before serving.

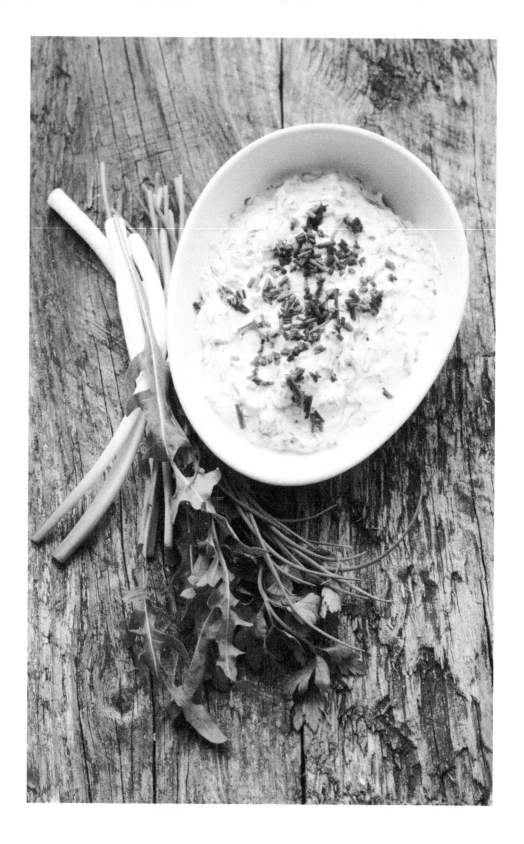

Onion and Herb Dip

SERVES 8

▸ *CALORIES PER SERVING* **58** // *SODIUM PER SERVING* **27MG**

Try this dip with raw vegetables or Vegetable Chips (page 197). It's also delicious spread on a sandwich, or used to flavor scrambled eggs. If you use yogurt instead of sour cream, stir in 1–2 tablespoons of crème fraîche for a little extra richness that doesn't break the bank calorie-wise. If you use a food processor to chop the onion, drain off the any excess liquid before adding it to the dip. Chopping the onion by hand is preferable for best results. This recipe is infinitely adaptable—consider adding one of the delicious optional ingredients to really up the wow factor.

....

2 cups reduced-fat sour cream or nonfat plain yogurt

1 bunch green onions, green and white parts sliced thin

1 cup finely chopped yellow onion

½ cup chopped parsley leaves

½ teaspoon cayenne pepper

Freshly ground pepper

Optional additions:

1 (6-ounce) can crabmeat, drained and picked over

6–7 chopped sun-dried tomatoes

1 cup chopped watercress

2 tablespoons freshly squeezed lemon juice

1 tablespoon crumbled blue cheese

Dill or cilantro leaves (instead of parsley)

....

1. Combine the sour cream, green onions, yellow onion, parsley, and cayenne in a medium bowl and mix well. Season with pepper. Refrigerate the dip for at least 1 hour to let the flavors blend before serving.

Roasted Red Pepper Dip

SERVES 4

▶ *CALORIES PER SERVING* **111** // *SODIUM PER SERVING* **32MG**

The simple technique of roasting peppers is the essence of this recipe. It can be mixed with light sour cream for a dip, but is is also a perfect sauce to spoon over grilled chicken or fish, add to mayonnaise for sandwiches, or simply toss with hot whole-wheat pasta. Serve the dip with fresh vegetables, Vegetable Chips (page 197), or toasted whole-wheat pita triangles.

5 large red bell peppers, halved, seeded, and de-ribbed

½ small jalapeño pepper, halved, seeded, and de-ribbed

1 tablespoon balsamic vinegar

1 tablespoon extra-virgin olive oil

1 teaspoon chopped garlic

Freshly ground pepper

3 tablespoons low-fat milk

2 teaspoons all-purpose flour

1 teaspoon cornstarch

¾ cup light sour cream

1. Preheat the broiler.

2. Slice the bell pepper and jalapeño halves in half again. Press the pepper pieces in your palm to flatten them. Place the peppers skin up in a single layer on a rimmed baking sheet. Broil 4–5 inches from the heat for 5–10 minutes, or until the skins are charred and flaking.

3. Immediately transfer the peppers to a bowl or paper bag and seal tightly. Let sit for 30 minutes while the steam loosens the skins.

4. When cool, peel the skins off completely, holding the peppers under cold running water to help the process along, if necessary. Transfer the peppers to the bowl of a food processor or a blender.

5. Add the balsamic vinegar, oil, and garlic, and process until the mixture is completely smooth. Season with pepper. The sauce can be used on meat or pasta.

6. For a dip, whisk together the milk, flour, and cornstarch in a small bowl until well combined. Add the sour cream and stir well. Add this mixture to the pureed pepper mixture and process until well combined. Add 1–2 tablespoons water as needed to achieve the desired consistency and flavor. Refrigerate for at least 1 hour to let the flavors blend before serving.

Spicy Oil-Roasted Chickpeas

SERVES 4

▶ *CALORIES PER SERVING* **233** // *SODIUM PER SERVING* **376MG**

Give chickpeas a crunchy exterior and they become extremely addictive. If you are going to have a "bad" snacking habit, chickpeas are a lot better than most. A serving of chickpeas is half the daily fiber required for the adults. Add in the copper, calcium, potassium, and iron (26 percent of your daily needs) and you can't afford not to eat these delicious legumes. Note that the dried chickpeas need to be soaked overnight, so be sure to plan ahead when making this recipe.

3 cups dried chickpeas, soaked in water overnight

4 cups white vinegar

2 tablespoons extra-virgin olive oil

1 teaspoon coarse sea salt (optional)

1 teaspoon cayenne pepper

1 teaspoon lemon zest

½ teaspoon paprika

1. Preheat the oven to 400° F.

2. Drain the chickpeas. In a large saucepan over medium-high heat, bring the vinegar to a boil. Add the chickpeas and return to a boil. Watch closely and as soon as the liquid begins to boil, remove the pan from the heat and let the chickpeas sit in the hot vinegar for 30 minutes. Drain the chickpeas, discarding the liquid, and then dry completely on paper towels.

3. Whisk together the oil, salt, cayenne, lemon zest, and paprika in a large bowl. Add the chickpeas to the oil mixture, toss well to coat, then spread in a single layer on a rimmed baking sheet or shallow roasting pan. Roast for about 45 minutes, checking the chickpeas every few minutes starting at the 30 minutes, to keep them from burning. Let cool and serve.

Homemade Hummus with Crudités

SERVES 8

▸ *CALORIES PER SERVING* **141** // *SODIUM PER SERVING* **282MG**

Hummus dip is so simple to make at home, you may feel a bit sheepish having ever bought it. This is a basic platform recipe; play with the flavors in the dip the same way you would vary what you dip into it. Try kalamata olives, a teaspoon of chopped capers, sun-dried tomatoes, pistachios, roasted garlic, cilantro, or parsley in future batches. See the list of dipping options and the surprising range of sodium levels and calories in each. Hummus can safely be left at room temperature, and you'll be amazed by who eats raw vegetables as they pass by.

1 (15-ounce) can low-sodium chickpeas, half of the liquid reserved

2 garlic cloves

3 tablespoons freshly squeezed lemon juice

2 tablespoons extra-virgin olive oil, plus more for drizzling

Ground white pepper

Assorted vegetables, for dipping

1. In a food processor, combine the chickpeas with their reserved liquid, the garlic, lemon juice, and oil, and season with white pepper. Process until smooth. Transfer the hummus to a small bowl and drizzle with a little more oil.

2. Place the bowl in the middle of a large platter and arrange a variety of vegetables around it.

Herbed Deviled Eggs

SERVES 6

▶ *CALORIES PER SERVING* **225** // *SODIUM PER SERVING* **180MG**

Almost everyone in America loves deviled eggs—it's the classic potluck and holiday favorite. Luckily for cooks, there are countless additions to deviled eggs that make them really sing. Experiment until you find your very favorite combination. Add a few tablespoons of finely chopped celery or red bell pepper, use a flavored mayonnaise, or play with different herbs and spices.

12 large hard-boiled eggs
3 tablespoons reduced-fat mayonnaise
1 tablespoon mustard
1 tablespoon finely minced onion
1 tablespoon finely chopped dill
1 teaspoon unseasoned rice vinegar
Freshly ground pepper
Paprika, for garnish

1. Peel the eggs carefully. Slice them in half lengthwise and scoop the yolk into a medium bowl. Set the egg whites aside.

2. Add the mayonnaise, mustard, onion, dill, and vinegar to the egg yolks and mix with a fork until smooth. Season with pepper and adjust the flavor as needed.

3. Using a tablespoon or melon baller, scoop a small round of the egg yolk mixture and press carefully into an egg white. Repeat until all the egg whites are filled. Arrange the eggs on a platter, sprinkle with paprika, and serve.

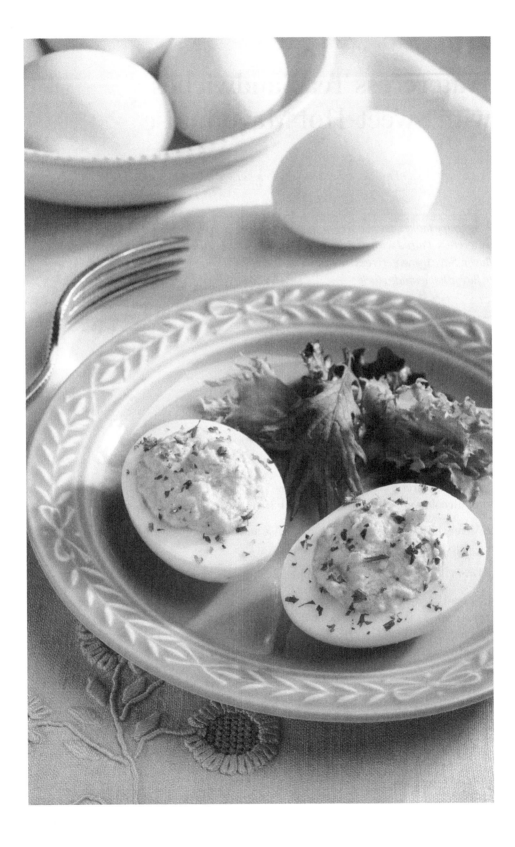

Watercress Tea Sandwiches with Sweet-Hot Mayonnaise

SERVES 8

▶ *CALORIES PER SERVING* **122** // *SODIUM PER SERVING* **118MG**

This recipe makes use of a technique to soften the overwhelming peppery taste of watercress. Paired with a sweet-hot mayonnaise, this little sandwich delivers big flavor. Save the watercress stems in a sealable plastic bag in the freezer and use later to flavor homemade stock.

1 cup stemmed watercress leaves
2 tablespoons white vinegar
Cold water
¼ cup reduced-fat mayonnaise
2 tablespoons honey
Hot sauce, to taste
8 thin slices whole-wheat bread

1. Put the watercress leaves in a large bowl. Add the vinegar and fill the bowl to the top with cold water. Let the leaves sit for 30 minutes to soften the peppery flavor.

2. Meanwhile, stir together the mayonnaise and honey and season to taste with hot sauce.

3. Drain the watercress and pat completely dry with paper towels.

4. Spread the mayonnaise mixture on all the bread slices. Layer a few watercress leaves on 4 of the slices, top each with a second slice, and trim the crusts off. Cut the sandwiches diagonally twice, making 4 small triangles. Arrange the sandwiches on a plate and serve.

Cilantro-Avocado Tea Sandwiches

SERVES 8

▶ *CALORIES PER SERVING* **412** // *SODIUM PER SERVING* **308MG**

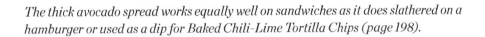

The thick avocado spread works equally well on sandwiches as it does slathered on a hamburger or used as a dip for Baked Chili-Lime Tortilla Chips (page 198).

2 ripe Hass avocados, cut into chunks
2 shallots, coarsely chopped
½ cup coarsely chopped cilantro leaves
Juice of 1 to 2 lemons
1 tablespoon extra-virgin olive oil
½ cup alfalfa sprouts
8 thin slices whole-wheat bread

1. Combine the avocados, shallots, cilantro, lemon juice, and oil in a food processor or blender and process until smooth. For a chunkier spread, mash the mixture with a fork.

2. Spread the mixture about a ½ inch thick on a slice of bread and top with 2 tablespoons of the sprouts. Top with a second slice and trim the crusts off. Cut the sandwich diagonally twice, making 4 small triangles. Repeat with the remaining bread, avocado spread, and sprouts. Arrange the sandwiches on a platter and serve.

Simple Lobster Tea Sandwiches

SERVES 8

▸ *CALORIES PER SERVING* **101** // *SODIUM PER SERVING* **324MG**

This is not your mother's mayonnaise-soaked lobster roll stuffing, although preparing lobster that way can be really good too. Here, a little unsalted butter, lemon juice, and parsley lightly flavors the lobster meat piled on a piece of toast.

1 (1-pound) cooked lobster, meat removed and diced
½ cup parsley leaves, chopped
2 tablespoons unsalted butter, melted
1 tablespoon freshly squeezed lemon juice
8 thin slices whole-wheat bread
Freshly ground pepper

1. Combine the lobster, parsley, butter, and lemon juice in a medium bowl and mix thoroughly.

2. Using a large glass as a guide, cut a round piece from the middle of each slice of bread and discard the trimmings. Toast the 8 rounds.

3. To assemble, pile a few tablespoons of lobster on each of the toast rounds and season with pepper. Arrange the sandwiches on a plate and serve.

Cucumber and Dill Tea Sandwiches

SERVES 8

▶ *CALORIES PER SERVING* **235** // *SODIUM PER SERVING* **300MG**

Pausing for a cup of tea and tiny sandwich at four o'clock not only makes sense energy-wise, it adds a moment for civility and pleasure on the most hectic of days. These tea sandwiches are small—this is just a little afternoon pick-me-up. Tradition calls for white bread, but whole grain is much healthier, so follow what's best for your heart.

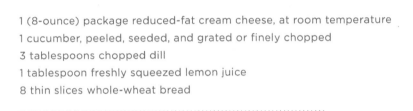

1 (8-ounce) package reduced-fat cream cheese, at room temperature
1 cucumber, peeled, seeded, and grated or finely chopped
3 tablespoons chopped dill
1 tablespoon freshly squeezed lemon juice
8 thin slices whole-wheat bread

1. Put the cream cheese in a medium bowl. Blot any excess moisture from the cucumber; then add it to the bowl along with the dill and lemon juice. Stir thoroughly to combine.

2. Spread a few tablespoons of the mixture on one slice of bread, top with another slice, and trim the crusts off. Cut the sandwich diagonally twice, making 4 small triangles. Repeat with the remaining bread and cucumber spread. Arrange the sandwiches on a plate and serve.

Shrimp and Mango "Ceviche"

SERVES 4

▶ *CALORIES PER SERVING* **96** // *SODIUM PER SERVING* **52MG**

Ceviche comes from Central and South America and is made in as many ways as there are home cooks. Traditionally, the seafood is not actually cooked, but instead marinated in acidic lemon or lime juice, which transforms it from translucent to opaque. In this version, the shrimp are cooked so this isn't a true ceviche, but it can safely be left sitting out at room temperature for parties.

1 pound small shrimp, cooked, peeled, and deveined

2 mangos, peeled and diced

1 medium red onion, chopped

1 red bell pepper, seeded and diced

1 jalapeño pepper, seeded and thinly sliced

½ cup chopped cilantro leaves

Juice of 2–3 limes

Freshly ground pepper

Boston or red leaf lettuce leaves

1. Combine the shrimp, mangoes, onion, bell pepper, jalapeño, cilantro, and lime juice in a medium bowl and stir well to combine. Season with pepper. Cover with plastic wrap and refrigerate for at least 2 hours, but preferably 4 hours.

2. To serve, line martini or wine glasses with lettuce leaves and spoon the shrimp mixture on top.

Turkey Mozzarella Shooters

SERVES 8

▸ *CALORIES PER SERVING* **263** // *SODIUM PER SERVING* **44MG***

Lean ground turkey is wrapped around spiced bocconcini and fried for a satisfying explosion of melted cheese halfway through each bite. Serve as finger food or with seafood forks or toothpicks.

1 pound lean ground turkey

1 large egg, beaten

1 teaspoon ground sage

Freshly ground pepper

10–16 ounces bocconcini in oil and herbs

2 tablespoons canola oil

1. Put the turkey, egg, and sage in a medium bowl and season with pepper. Mix with clean hands until the egg is thoroughly combined with the turkey.

2. Slice the bocconcini in half. Form a small handful of the turkey mixture into a patty or ball and work a bocconcini into the center, sealing the turkey around it. Repeat until all the turkey and bocconcini have been used.

3. Heat the oil in a large skillet over medium-high heat. When the oil is hot, fry the turkey balls in batches until cooked through, 3–5 minutes. Transfer the balls to paper towels to drain, and then serve immediately.

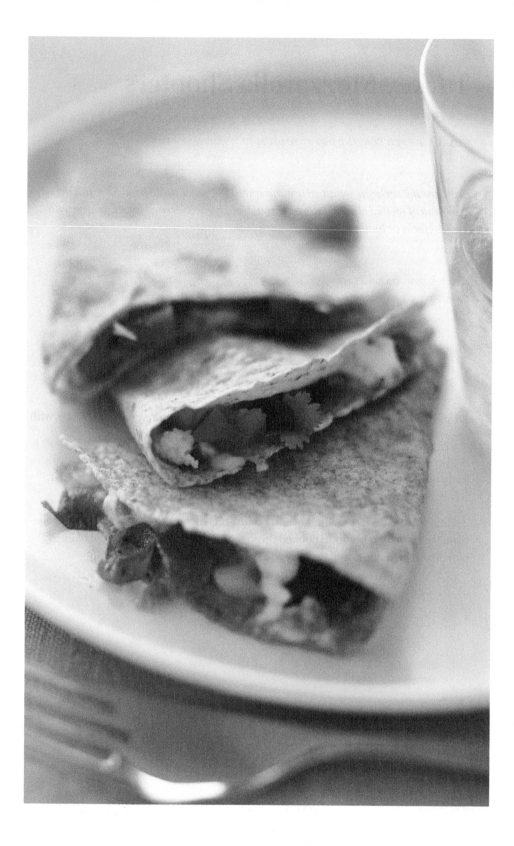

Tiny Turkey Quesadillas

SERVES 4

▶ *CALORIES PER SERVING* **247** // *SODIUM PER SERVING* **146MG**

This recipe makes simple quesadillas, softened in a pan and piled high with deli turkey, tomatoes, avocado, and sprouts. Emmentaler is a spectacular melting cheese that is lower in sodium than most other cheeses.

1 avocado, thinly sliced
Juice of 1 lemon
2 whole-wheat tortillas
2 slices Emmentaler or other Swiss cheese
4–8 extra-thin slices deli turkey
2 Roma tomatoes, thinly sliced lengthwise
2 ounces alfalfa sprouts
Freshly ground pepper

1. Put the avocado in a small bowl and toss well with the lemon juice to keep it from turning brown. Set out all the other ingredients on a platter for quick quesadilla assembly.

2. Heat a nonstick skillet over medium-high heat. Add the first tortilla and brown one side quickly, about 30 seconds. Flip it over and place a slice of cheese on one half of the tortilla. When the cheese begins to soften and melt, transfer the tortilla to a plate.

3. Working quickly, layer half of the turkey, tomatoes, sprouts, and avocado on top of the cheese. Season with pepper. Fold the tortilla over the filling and secure with toothpicks. Cut the quesadilla into 2–4 wedges. Repeat with the second tortilla and serve.

Lemon-Glazed Tiny Drumsticks

SERVES 6

▶ *CALORIES PER SERVING* **177** // *SODIUM PER SERVING* **71MG**

You may unleash rabid monsters when you set out these little chicken legs redolent of lemon and herbs. Consider making a double batch to avoid battles at the table.

1 cup freshly squeezed lemon juice
¼ cup fresh oregano leaves
3 tablespoons honey
Freshly ground pepper
12 small chicken drumsticks, rinsed in cold water and patted dry

1. Whisk together the lemon juice, oregano, and honey in a small bowl. Season with pepper. Pour the mixture into a large, sealable plastic bag. Add the drumsticks to the bag, seal, and shake until the chicken is well coated in marinade. Refrigerate for at least 1 hour.

2. Preheat the oven to 375º F.

3. Transfer the drumsticks to a rimmed baking sheet. Bake for 50–60 minutes, or until the meat almost falls from the bone. Serve the drumsticks hot, at room temperature, or cold. You can use the marinade as a dipping sauce by boiling it over medium-high heat until thickened.

Thai Pork in Lettuce Wraps

SERVES 4

▶ *CALORIES PER SERVING* **280** // *SODIUM PER SERVING* **603MG**

Southeast Asian cooking has a tradition of using lettuce leaves as edible packaging for delicious meats and vegetables. Simply scoop the filling into a leaf, roll it up, and voilà, you've gone mobile. The wrapper is both delicious and happily leaves no waste behind. This dish can be made with lean ground turkey or chicken instead of pork, if desired. It's not the Thai way, but using turkey will save 130 calories and using chicken saves 146.

1½ pounds lean ground pork
2 shallots, minced
2 garlic cloves, minced
1 jalapeño pepper, seeded and minced
1 tablespoon vegetable oil
½ cup chopped cilantro leaves
½ cup chopped mint leaves
½ cup chopped basil leaves
Juice of 1 lime
1 tablespoon reduced-sodium fish sauce
1 teaspoon light brown sugar
1 teaspoon chili sauce
8 red leaf or Boston lettuce leaves, washed and dried

1. In a large bowl, combine the pork, shallots, garlic, and jalapeño, and stir well.

2. Heat the oil in a large skillet over medium-high heat. When the oil is hot, add the pork mixture and break apart the meat as much as possible with a spatula. Reduce the heat to medium and cook through, but do not brown the pork. Remove the pan from the heat.

3. Whisk together the cilantro, mint, basil, lime juice, fish sauce, brown sugar, and chili sauce in a medium bowl until thoroughly combined.

4. Stir the herb mixture into the pan and mix thoroughly with the pork. Let cool slightly before serving with the lettuce.

DASH Meatballs

SERVES 8

▶ *CALORIES PER SERVING* **416** // *SODIUM PER SERVING* **263MG**

Back in the 1960s, hostesses all over the world lit Sterno cans beneath their chafing dishes to keep the meatballs warm through the cocktail hour. No need to worry about that here. These meatballs will be gone long before they have a chance to become cold. Remember, toothpicks are essential for meatball consumption.

2 large eggs
1 cup breadcrumbs
2 pounds lean ground beef
Freshly ground pepper
⅓ cup chopped onions
1 cup jellied cranberry sauce
½ cup orange marmalade
½ cup low-sodium chicken broth
1 tablespoon minced jalapeño pepper

1. Preheat the oven to 350° F.

2. In a medium bowl, beat the eggs and 4 tablespoons water together. Add the breadcrumbs and stir well.

3. In a large bowl, break apart the ground beef and season it with plenty of pepper. Add the onions and egg mixture to the ground beef and stir well to combine.

4. Form the mixture into 1-inch round balls and place in a single layer on a rimmed baking sheet. Bake for 20–25 minutes, or until cooked through.

5. In a large Dutch oven, deep skillet, or heavy-bottomed pot, combine the cranberry sauce, marmalade, and chicken broth. Season with pepper and mix thoroughly. Add the meatballs to the pan and gently stir to coat the meatballs evenly with sauce.

6. Bring the sauce to a gentle simmer over medium heat; then reduce to low and cook the meatballs for 30 minutes. Serve immediately with toothpicks and napkins.

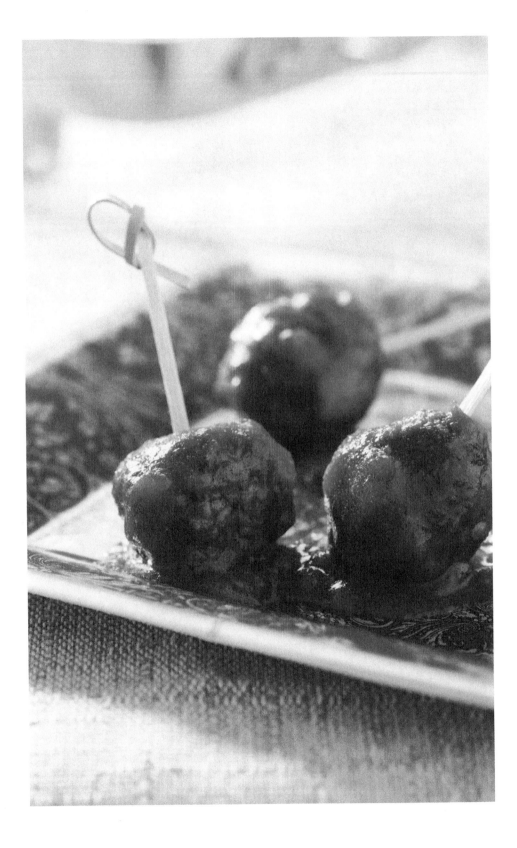

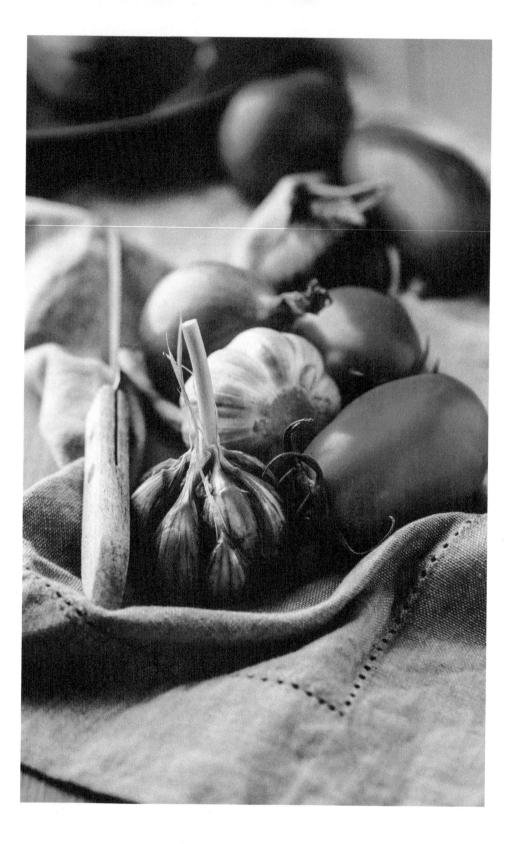

CHAPTER FIFTEEN

DASH Dinners

- Quick Vegetarian Ramen Noodle Soup

- Coconut Fish Stew

- Turkey Chili with Black Beans

- Vegetable Beef Stew

- Creamy Beans and Greens

- Bulgur with Vegetables and Goat Cheese

- Layered Vegetable Casserole

- Kale and Tomatoes on Whole-Wheat Pasta

- Pasta with Basil or Cilantro Pesto

- Portobello Stroganoff over Egg Noodles

- Vegetable Lasagna

- Turkey Bolognese

- Spicy Tofu Stir-Fry

- Pan-Seared Whitefish on Lemony Quinoa

- Perfect Pan-Seared Fish

- Shrimp with Jalapeño-Orange Sauce over Pasta

- Louisiana Shrimp Boil

- Turkey and Rice–Stuffed Peppers

- Lemon-Scented Chicken Kebabs on Saffron Rice

- Panko-Crusted Chicken Strips with Apricot Dipping Sauce

- Best Practices Roast Chicken

- Chicken Breasts with Citrus and Chili Sauce on Coconut Rice

- Chicken Breasts with Mushroom Sauce on Wild Rice

- Chicken Breasts with Mango-Rosemary Sauce on Brown Rice

- The Winemaker's Feast

- Grilled Pork Tenderloin with Garlic and Herbs

- Boneless Pork Chops with Curried Apples

- Scottish Meatloaf

- Argentinean-Style Flank Steak

- Pot Roast with Sweet Potatoes, Peas, and Onions

Quick Vegetarian Ramen Noodle Soup

SERVES 4

▶ *CALORIES PER SERVING* **250** // *SODIUM PER SERVING* **458MG**

Spend a few minutes cutting up vegetables for this nutritious weekday soup. It comes together in minutes and leaves you satisfied all through the night.

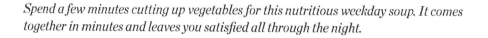

1 (8-ounce) package ramen noodles
1 quart low-sodium vegetable broth
1 (15-ounce) can diced tomatoes, drained
1 cup diced zucchini
1 orange bell pepper, seeded and diced
1 carrot, diced
2 garlic cloves, chopped
1 tablespoon low-sodium soy sauce
½ cup julienned zucchini, for garnish (optional)

1. Cook the noodles according to the pacakge directions, drain, and set aside.

2. In a large stockpot over medium-high heat, combine the broth, tomatoes, diced zucchini, bell pepper, carrot, and garlic.

3. Boil the vegetables for 5–10 minutes, or until tender.

4. Remove the pot from the heat and add the noodles and soy sauce. Ladle the soup into 4 bowls and serve immediately, garnished with the julienned zucchini, if desired.

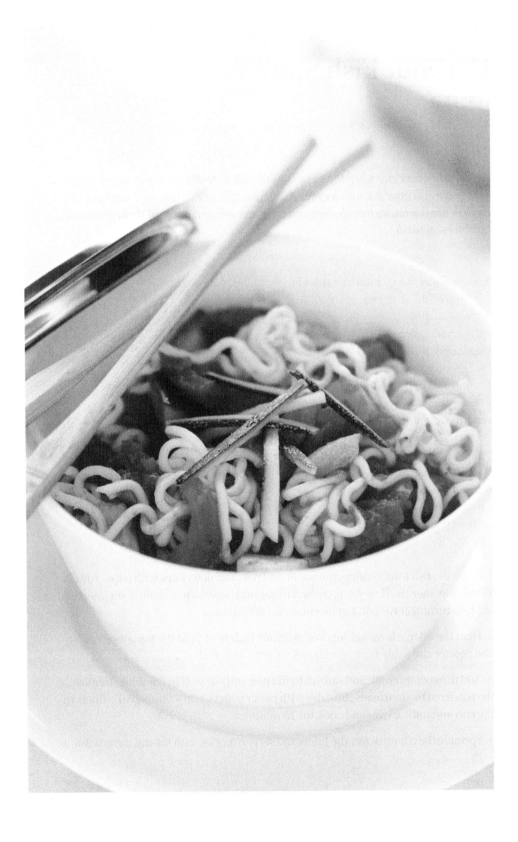

Coconut Fish Stew

SERVES 4

▶ *CALORIES PER SERVING* **393** // *SODIUM PER SERVING* **86MG**

Eat this stew over rice when the snow is piled high outside and daydream about the Caribbean. Coconut is a wonder food full of good fat, potassium, and magnesium. Its flesh also increases metabolism and the water inside it is one of the best human hydrators on earth.

2 pounds fish fillets, such as sea bass, trout, cod, tilapia, salmon, swordfish, or shrimp

Juice of 2 limes

1 clove garlic, smashed

1 teaspoon ground cumin

1 teaspoon paprika

2 tablespoons extra-virgin olive oil

6 Roma tomatoes, quartered

1 cup diced onion

1 cup diced red bell pepper

1 (14-ounce) can full-fat coconut milk

½ teaspoon saffron powder

¼ cup finely chopped cilantro leaves

Lemon wedges, for serving

Cooked rice

1. Rinse the fish fillets under cold water and pat completely dry with paper towels. Whisk together the lime juice, garlic, cumin, and paprika in a shallow dish and add the fish, turning it to coat. Let marinate for 30 minutes.

2. Heat the oil in a large skillet over medium-high heat. Add the tomatoes, onion, and pepper and sauté for 5–8 minutes, or until softened.

3. Add the coconut milk and saffron to the pan and stir well to combine. Remove the fish from the marinade, blot dry with paper towels, and submerge the fillets in the coconut milk. Cover and cook for 15 minutes.

4. Sprinkle the cilantro over the fillets and serve over rice with the quartered lemons.

Turkey Chili with Black Beans

SERVES 6

▶ *CALORIES PER SERVING* **353** // *SODIUM PER SERVING* **311MG**

Ground spices do most of the heavy lifting flavor-wise in this turkey chili, transforming the tomatoes, vegetables, beans, and meat into a big pot of nuanced flavor. Some favorite additions to serve alongside the chili include shredded cheddar cheese, sour cream, and chopped cilantro. Put the garnishes in small bowls and let diners help themselves.

1 tablespoon extra-virgin olive oil
2 pounds lean ground turkey
1 large onion, finely chopped
1 cup finely chopped yellow bell pepper
2 tablespoons minced garlic
1 (28-ounce) can crushed tomatoes
1 (14.5-ounce) can reduced-sodium chicken broth
2 cups dried black beans, soaked in water overnight and drained
2 tablespoons chili powder
1 teaspoon paprika
1 teaspoon dried oregano
1 teaspoon ground cumin
Freshly ground pepper

1. In a large stockpot, heat the oil over medium-high heat. When the oil is hot, add the turkey and cook, stirring, until just browned. Add the onion, bell pepper, and garlic and continue to cook until the vegetables are softened, about 5 minutes.

2. Add 4 cups water, the tomatoes, chicken broth, black beans, chili powder, paprika, oregano, cumin, and pepper to the pot and increase the heat to high. When the chili begins to boil, reduce the heat to maintain a low simmer and cook for about 30 minutes, stirring frequently. The chili is ready when the beans are firm to the bite and creamy inside. Serve immediately.

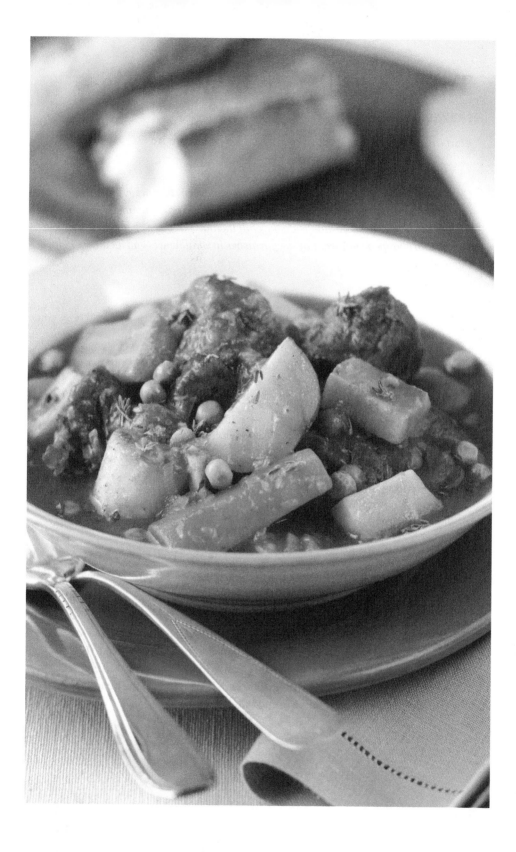

Vegetable Beef Stew

SERVES 4

▶ *CALORIES PER SERVING* **439** // *SODIUM PER SERVING* **475MG**

Beef broth is the perfect medium to deliver hearty, tender vegetables. The small amount of meat used here is mostly for flavor. This stove-top recipe is also perfect for a slow cooker: Nothing beats walking into a house that smells like dinner. The slow cooker method cooks the meat slowly overnight on low heat, then adds the vegetables in the morning, and the stew continues to cook on low all day.

1 (14.5-ounce) can low-sodium beef broth

½ pound beef stew meat, cut into 1-inch or smaller cubes

1 large onion, diced

2 garlic cloves, coarsely chopped

½ pound small new potatoes, cut into wedges

1 cup chopped carrots

1 cup frozen peas, thawed

2 to 3 sprigs rosemary, leaves removed and chopped, plus additional for garnish

Freshly ground pepper

Juice of 1 lemon

1. Place a large stockpot over medium-high heat and add the beef broth, beef, onion, garlic, and enough water to fill the pot one-third full. Bring to a boil; then reduce the heat to medium and simmer for at least 1 hour, preferably 2 hours. The longer the base simmers, the richer the stew will be.

2. Add the potatoes, carrots, peas, rosemary, and enough water to fill the pot two-thirds full. Simmer for another 45 minutes. Season the stew with pepper and lemon juice. Divide the stew among 4 bowls and serve immediately, garnished with additional rosemary, if desired.

Creamy Beans and Greens

SERVES 4

▶ *CALORIES PER SERVING* **265** // *SODIUM PER SERVING* **113MG**

Healthy and simple, this is almost like thick porridge for the nights when you need comfort and warmth. Beans are full of fiber, iron, and other minerals. Easy to prepare, they can go with even more healthy ingredients such as leafy greens, root vegetables, and herbs. Keep beans in your pantry and often on your dinner table.

1 tablespoon extra-virgin olive oil, plus more for drizzling
1 pound dried white kidney beans, soaked overnight and drained
1 small onion, chopped
2 cups low-sodium vegetable broth
2 to 3 large handfuls arugula or spinach, whole or shredded
Freshly ground pepper

1. In a large stockpot, heat the oil over medium-high heat. When the oil is hot, add the onion and cook, stirring occasionally, until soft, about 5 minutes. Add the vegetable broth.

2. Add the beans to the pot. Add water, if needed, to just cover the beans. Increase the heat to high and bring to a boil; then reduce the heat to maintain a simmer. Cook the beans, stirring occasionally, until very soft and creamy, at least 1 hour. Remove the pot from the heat.

3. Using a potato masher or the back of a wooden spoon, smash half of the beans so the texture is partially puréed with some whole beans.

4. Return the pot to the stove and place over medium-low heat. Add the arugula or spinach and stir until incorporated and warmed through. Ladle the beans into 4 bowls, season with pepper, and drizzle with a little oil. Serve immediately.

Bulgur with Vegetables and Goat Cheese

SERVES 4

▶ *CALORIES PER SERVING* **317** // *SODIUM PER SERVING* **18MG**

Bulgur is a delicious wheat grain and the perfect backdrop for vegetables and cheese. It's ready in just 20 minutes and can be combined with everything from roast chicken to deep-fried tofu for an earthy, satisfying meal.

2 cups cherry tomatoes, halved

1 cup broccoli florets, blanched

½ cup coarsely chopped red bell pepper

2 shallots, minced

½ cup chopped parsley leaves

2 tablespoons red wine vinegar

2 tablespoons extra-virgin olive oil

1 cup bulgur, cooked according to package directions

1 ounce fresh goat cheese, crumbled

1. In a large bowl, combine the tomatoes, broccoli, bell pepper, shallots, and parsley. Add the vinegar and oil, and toss well to combine. Add the cooked bulgur and toss again.

2. Sprinkle the goat cheese over the top and serve in large bowls.

Layered Vegetable Casserole

SERVES 4

▶ *CALORIES PER SERVING* **272** // *SODIUM PER SERVING* **199MG**

In a casserole or deep pie dish, layer vegetables with spices and oil and let them slowly roast into a slightly sweet, completely delectable casserole. Just one vegetarian meal a week does wonders for reducing your carbon footprint, as well as your sodium intake. Be sure to check the label on the mozzarella carefully: sodium contents vary wildly.

1 eggplant, thinly sliced

3 tablespoons extra-virgin olive oil

1–2 tablespoons dried oregano, divided

½ pound unsalted fresh mozzarella, cut into 1-inch cubes

2 zucchini, thinly sliced

1 medium yellow squash, thinly sliced

1 pint cherry tomatoes, halved

Kernels from 2 ears corn

1 tablespoon grated Parmesan cheese

Freshly ground pepper

1. Preheat the oven to 400° F.

2. In a large baking dish, arrange the eggplant slices in the bottom, drizzled with ½ tablespoon of the oil. Sprinkle with a bit of the oregano and dot with some of the mozzarella cubes. Repeat this layering with the zucchini, squash, tomatoes, and corn until all the vegetables have been used.

3. Sprinkle the Parmesan on top, season with pepper, and bake for 1 hour. Serve immediately.

Kale and Tomatoes on Whole-Wheat Pasta

SERVES 6

▶ *CALORIES PER SERVING* **498** // *SODIUM PER SERVING* **59MG**

Like broccoli or sweet potato, kale is so good for you, you should work it into your diet whenever possible. This quick and easy pasta sauce—with toasted almonds added for crunch—is as simple as it is packed with great nutrition.

1 pound whole-wheat spaghetti or other pasta

2 tablespoons extra-virgin olive oil, plus more for drizzling

1 large red onion, thinly sliced and rings separated

2 garlic cloves, minced

1 large bunch kale, stems removed and torn into bite-sized pieces

2 pints grape tomatoes, halved

⅓ cup slivered almonds, toasted

1. Cook the pasta according to package instructions and drain, reserving ¼ cup cooking water. Transfer the pasta to a large serving bowl and drizzle with a little oil.

2. Heat the olive oil over medium-high heat in a large skillet. Add the onion and garlic and cook until they soften and turn translucent, about 5 minutes. Add the kale to the pan, stir well, and cook for 2 to 3 minutes. Add the tomatoes and the reserved ¼ cup cooking water, and cook for 2 to 3 minutes, or until the tomatoes begin to release their juices.

3. Pour the tomato sauce over the pasta, sprinkle with the almonds, and toss thoroughly to incorporate. Serve immediately.

Pasta with Basil or Cilantro Pesto

SERVES 4

▶ *CALORIES PER SERVING* **488** // *SODIUM PER SERVING* **100MG**

Either of these no-cook pesto sauces turn pasta into a heavenly tasting dish that evokes spring. Parmesan cheese is high in sodium but a little goes a long way: each diner gets less than ½ teaspoon per serving. Use basil or cilantro from your own garden, and this dish improves tenfold—there's nothing better than freshly picked herbs.

1 pound whole-wheat pasta

2 cups basil or cilantro leaves, packed tight

¼ cup pine nuts (for basil) or ¼ cup walnuts or pecans (for cilantro)

2 garlic cloves

¼ cup grated Parmesan cheese

⅔ cup extra-virgin olive oil

1. Bring a large pot of water to a boil for cooking the pasta.

2. While the water is heating, put the basil or cilantro, nuts, and garlic into a food processor and process for about 1 minute, then add the Parmesan. Drizzle the olive oil through the feed tube in a steady stream and process just until the mixture forms a smooth paste.

3. Cook the pasta according to package directions. Drain in a colander.

4. Return the pasta to the cooking pot, add 2–3 heaping tablespoons of the pesto, and toss thoroughly to coat. Serve the pasta warm or at room temperature. Any remaining pesto can be stored in the refrigerator in an airtight container for 1 week.

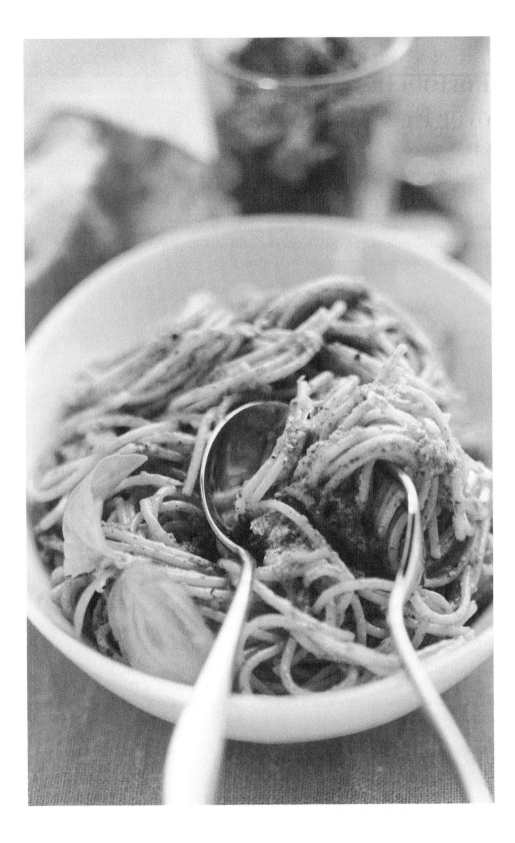

Portobello Stroganoff over Egg Noodles

6 SERVINGS

▸ *CALORIES PER SERVING* **318** // *SODIUM PER SERVING* **79MG**

Portobello mushrooms are thick and meaty, and egg noodles are rich-tasting and have almost no sodium. This dish is delicious and comforting. Note that all-purpose flour thickens the sauce better than whole-wheat flour.

3 tablespoons canola oil

1 large onion, finely chopped

1 pound portobello mushroom caps, thickly sliced

1 (12-ounce) package egg noodles

2 cups low-sodium vegetable broth

2 cups reduced-fat sour cream

3 tablespoons all-purpose flour

½ cup chopped parsley leaves

1. In a large skillet, heat the oil over medium heat. Add the onion and cook until very soft, but not brown, about 8 minutes. Increase the heat to medium-high and add the mushrooms, cooking them until they become soft and turn dark brown. Transfer the mixture to a medium bowl and set aside.

2. Bring a pot of water to a boil and cook the noodles according to the package directions. Drain and transfer them to a large serving bowl.

3. Meanwhile, in the same skillet used to cook the mushrooms, boil the broth vigorously, reducing it by one-third. Return the mushrooms to the pan and stir to combine.

4. In a small bowl, stir together the sour cream and flour. Whisk the mixture into the pan, stirring constantly as the the sauce thickens, 2–3 minutes. Pour the sauce over the noodles and sprinkle with the parsley. Serve immediately.

Vegetable Lasagna

SERVES 6

▶ *CALORIES PER SERVING* **520** // *SODIUM PER SERVING* **474MG**

The vegetables in this dish roast slowly in the oven and turn into a flavorful lasagna filling. Fresh mozzarella has far less salt than most cheeses, but it's too moist for lasagna. To counteract this, simply slice it and let it drain, uncovered, in the refrigerator overnight. The roasted vegetables, sauce, and ricotta mixture can all be made in advance and the lasagna assembled just before baking.

2 cups coarsely chopped zucchini

2 cups coarsely chopped yellow squash

2 cups peeled and coarsely chopped eggplant

2 tablespoons extra-virgin olive oil, plus more for drizzling

2 pounds Roma tomatoes, quartered

1 (14.5-ounce) can low-sodium, fat-free chicken broth

2 garlic cloves, smashed

1 (15-ounce) package part-skim ricotta cheese

2 large eggs, beaten

½ cup shredded basil leaves

2 tablespoons shredded Parmesan cheese

1 (16-ounce) package lasagna noodles

1 pound fresh unsalted mozzarella, sliced and dried overnight

1. Preheat the oven to 400° F.

2. Toss the zucchini, squash, and eggplant with the olive oil, adding more if needed to coat. Spread the vegetables in a single layer on rimmed baking sheets. Roast the vegetables for 1 hour, stirring once halfway through the cooking. Transfer the vegetables to a large bowl and set aside.

3. Put the tomatoes, broth, and garlic in a large saucepan and bring to a boil over high heat. Boil vigorously for 30 minutes. Let the tomatoes cool slightly; then process until smooth in a food process or blender. This is the lasagna sauce: If it's too thin, return the sauce to the pan and reduce over medium-high heat. If it's too thick, add a little water.

continued ▶

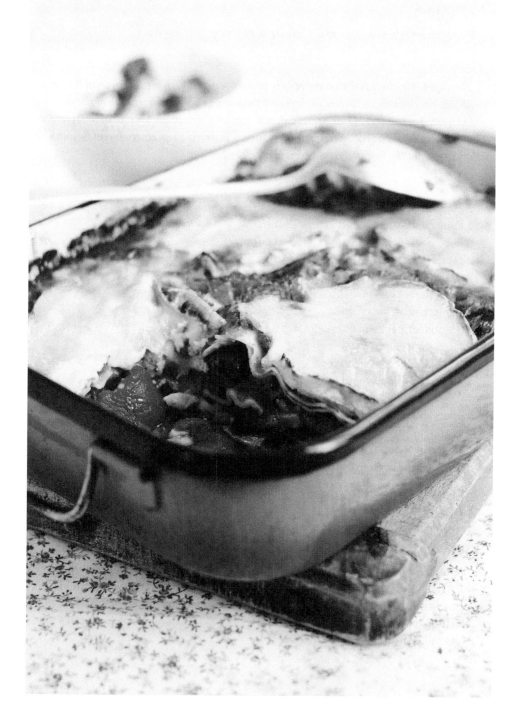

4. Put the ricotta in a large bowl with the eggs, basil, and Parmesan. Using an electric mixer or a whisk, whip the ricotta mixture until it is light and airy. Set aside.

5. Boil the noodles according to package directions. Drain and then drizzle with a little oil to keep the noodles from sticking together.

6. To assemble the lasagna, spread ½ cup sauce on the bottom of a large roasting pan. Put a single layer of lasagna noodles on the sauce. Spoon about ½ cup of the ricotta mixture over the noodles and spread evenly. Layer some roasted vegetables over the ricotta. Cut 1 mozzarella slice into 1-inch cubes and scatter over the vegetables. Put a second layer of lasagna noodles over the vegetables, then another layer of sauce. Continue layering the ricotta, vegetables, mozzarella, noodles, and sauce, ending with a layer of noodles topped with sauce. Scatter any remaining mozzarella cubes over the top, and bake for 1 hour. Let the lasagna rest for 10 minutes before serving.

Turkey Bolognese

SERVES 4

▸ *CALORIES PER SERVING* **316** // *SODIUM PER SERVING* **147MG**

Northern Italy gave the world this pasta sauce, in which meat is gently cooked in milk and then turned into a robust tomato sauce for pasta. This recipe uses ground turkey and requires a good 3 hours of cooking to reach a glorious state of perfection. This is what is meant by "slow food," and it is worth it.

2 tablespoons extra-virgin olive oil

1 large onion, finely diced

2 carrots, peeled and finely shredded

1 stalk celery, finely chopped

3 garlic cloves, minced

2 pounds lean ground turkey

1 cup red wine

1 cup low-fat milk

1 (28-ounce) can no-sodium crushed or diced tomatoes

1 tablespoon dried oregano

1 pound whole-wheat pasta

Grated Parmesan cheese, for garnish

1. Heat the oil in a large pot or deep skillet over medium-high heat. Add the onion, carrots, celery, and garlic. Reduce the heat to medium and cook the vegetables until softened, about 5 minutes.

2. Add the turkey to the pot, breaking it apart with a wooden spoon. Add the red wine, stir well, and increase the heat to maintain a gentle simmer, cooking the sauce until it is reduced by one-third. Add the milk and continue to simmer until the sauce is reduced again by one-third.

3. Add the tomatoes and oregano and gently simmer the sauce, stirring occasionally, over low heat for 3 hours. Watch for bubbles breaking the surface every so often in this slow simmer.

4. Near the end of cooking, boil the pasta according to the package directions. Drain and transfer to a large serving bowl. Pour the sauce over the top and sprinkle lightly with Parmesan. Toss well to combine and serve immediately.

Spicy Tofu Stir-Fry

SERVES 4

▶ *CALORIES PER SERVING* **265** // *SODIUM PER SERVING* **174MG**

Tofu is so tasty when the water is pressed and seasonings are pressed in. This recipe is quick, easy, and delicious and is a good base for creating new dishes. Serve this stir-fry with or without brown rice—it's plenty filling on its own.

1 pound firm tofu, drained well

3 teaspoons cornstarch, divided

3 tablespoons vegetable oil

1 red onion, thinly sliced and rings separated

1 red bell pepper, seeded and diced

1 green chile, seeded and diced

3 garlic cloves, diced

3 tablespoons white vinegar

1 teaspoon soy sauce

1 tablespoon brown sugar

1 tablespoon crushed red pepper flakes

1. Cut the tofu in half lengthwise, creating as much surface area as possible. Place the tofu on paper towels, layer more paper towels over it, and place a heavy pan or weighted plate on top to press out the water. Let drain for at least 1 hour.

2. Cut the tofu into cubes and toss in a medium bowl with 2 teaspoons of the cornstarch.

3. Heat the oil in a wok over medium-high heat. Add the tofu, onion, bell pepper, and chile and stir-fry until the vegetables are soft and the tofu is crunchy.

4. In a small bowl, whisk together ⅓ cup hot water, the remaining 1 teaspoon of cornstarch, the vinegar, soy sauce, brown sugar, and red pepper flakes until thoroughly combined. Pour the sauce into the wok and toss well to combine. Serve immediately.

Pan-Seared Whitefish on Lemony Quinoa

SERVES 4

▸ *CALORIES PER SERVING* **442** // *SODIUM PER SERVING* **84MG**

To cook this fish well, you want plenty of very hot oil in the pan to create the browned, crunchy exterior and cook the fillet through quickly. For a well-rounded meal, the nutty, lemony quinoa is full of calcium and potassium for your heart and a low calorie count for your waist.

1 to 1½ pounds white fish fillets
1 cup quinoa
Zest and juice of 1 lemon
½ cup chopped parsley leaves
2 tablespoons extra-virgin olive oil
1 tablespoon margarine

1. Rinse the fish fillets under cold running water and pat completely dry with paper towels. To create a crisp brown crust, the fish can have no trace of moisture when it hits the oil in the pan.

2. Put the quinoa in a fine-mesh strainer and place under cold running water for about 30 seconds, shaking occasionally. This step helps remove any bitterness. Bring 3 cups water to a boil in a medium pot. Add the quinoa and cook, stirring occasionally, for about 20 minutes, or until the water has been absorbed. Remove the pot from the heat and stir in the lemon zest and parsley.

3. Heat the olive oil and margarine in a large heavy-bottomed or cast-iron skillet. When it is very hot, add the fish fillets, skin side down, and cook for 1 to 4 minutes, depending on the thickness of the fillets. The fish will become opaque and appear flaky. Flip the fish over and cook for 1–4 minutes on the other side until done.

4. Spoon the quinoa onto 4 plates, lay the fish on top, sprinkle with lemon juice, and serve immediately.

Perfect Pan-Seared Fish

SERVES 4

▶ *CALORIES PER SERVING* **351** // *SODIUM PER SERVING* **110MG**

This searing technique is the same one used by fancy New York chefs when cooking fish. The secret is now yours. Fish is best cooked in a small skillet that holds just one fillet at a time. You can cook these quickly and hold them in a warm oven, but try to get two pans working at once. Remember, a cook is only as good as his or her ingredients. Fresh fish should have virtually no smell. Shop wisely and sniff everything you see.

4 firm white fish fillets, with skin
¼ cup canola oil, divided
Freshly ground pepper

1. Heat about ½ inch of oil in 2 skillets over medium-high heat until the oil is fiercely hot—at least 1 to 2 minutes.

2. Put the first fish fillet, skin side down, into the pan. Be careful: it will splatter. Cook until the skin is crispy and the flesh around the edges is translucent and cooked through. Flip the fish over carefully—a fish spatula is best for this, but a regular one will work if used with care. Cook the skinless side until the flesh is just translucent, 2–3 minutes. Season with pepper and serve immediately or keep warm until ready to serve.

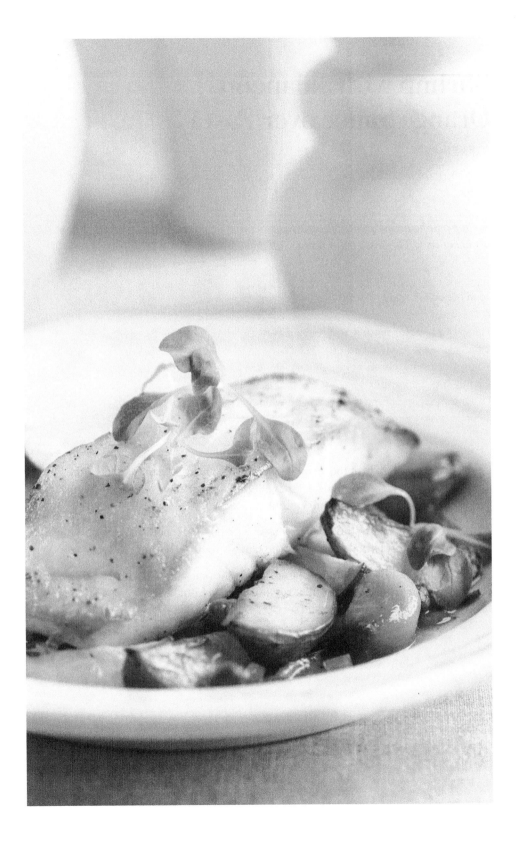

Shrimp with Jalapeño-Orange Sauce over Pasta

SERVES 4

▶ *CALORIES PER SERVING* **281** // *SODIUM PER SERVING* **102MG**

Shrimp pair beautifully with the sweetness of orange and the heat of tiny bits of pepper in between. The pasta helps soak up all the glorious juices in this dish.

1 tablespoon extra-virgin olive oil
4 shallots, finely diced
1 jalapeño pepper, seeded and finely diced
2 garlic cloves, finely diced
¾ cup freshly squeezed orange juice
Freshly ground pepper
1 pound medium shrimp, peeled and deveined
2 cups cooked angel hair pasta

1. In a medium skillet, heat the oil over medium-high heat. Add the shallots, jalapeño, and garlic, and reduce the heat to medium. Cook, stirring occasionally, until the vegetables are softened, about 5 minutes.

2. Add the orange juice to the pan and season with pepper. Increase the heat to high and bring to a vigorous boil. Cook until the sauce is reduced by one-third.

3. Reduce the heat to medium, add the shrimp to the pan, and toss well. As soon as the shrimp turn pink, 2–3 minutes, remove the pan from the heat. Spoon the shrimp and sauce over the pasta and serve.

Louisiana Shrimp Boil

SERVES 4

▸ *CALORIES PER SERVING* **230** // *SODIUM PER SERVING* **491MG**

This dish creates a party whenever you make it. There's no plates or silverware, just a huge platter on a table covered with newspaper. Have a roll of paper towels and some trash bags handy to keep things from getting too messy. The key to flavor here is how you spice the water. Don't use the commercial crab boils, as the sodium is too high. Besides, making your own seasoning combination is more fun, and soon you'll have a "secret family spice mixture" to brag about.

2 tablespoons extra-virgin olive oil

2 onions, thinly sliced

1 jalapeño pepper, seeded and thinly sliced

12 garlic cloves, peeled and halved

2 (1-inch) pieces ginger, peeled

12 whole cloves

12 black peppercorns

6 bay leaves, crushed

2 tablespoons coriander seed

2 tablespoons whole allspice

1 tablespoon hot sauce

4 ears corn, cut into thirds

1 pound small red or blue potatoes

2 pounds large shrimp, with their shells

2 lemons, cut into wedges

1. Heat the oil in a large stockpot over medium heat. Add the onions, jalapeño, garlic, and ginger, and cook until the vegetables are soft and translucent, 8–10 minutes.

2. Wrap the cloves, peppercorns, bay leaves, coriander, and allspice in cheesecloth or a very thin kitchen towel, and tie it into a little packet.

continued ▶

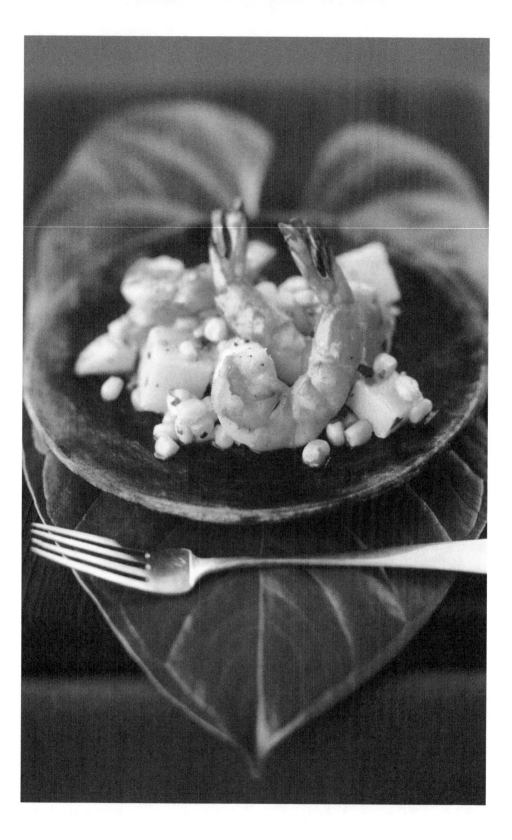

3. Add 3 quarts water, hot sauce, and the cheesecloth-wrapped spices to the pot. Increase the heat to high and bring to a rolling boil.

4. Add the corn and potatoes to the pot and cook until the potatoes are firm and can be pierced with a fork, 10–15 minutes. Add the shrimp and cook until just pink, about 3 minutes. Drain and then dump the entire contents of the pot onto a large platter. Serve with lemon wedges.

Turkey and Rice–Stuffed Peppers

SERVES 4

▶ *CALORIES PER SERVING* **300** // *SODIUM PER SERVING* **207MG**

This traditional stuffed pepper is filled with ground turkey, rice, mushrooms, garlic, and cumin. Each diner should get two halves. A nice big salad will round out the meal.

1½ pounds lean ground turkey
1 medium onion, chopped
2 garlic cloves, chopped
2 cups fat-free chicken broth, divided
¼ cup tomato sauce
1 teaspoon ground cumin
Freshly ground pepper
1 cup cooked brown rice
4 large red bell peppers, halved, seeded, and de-ribbed
¼ cup reduced-fat cheddar cheese
1 tablespoon chopped parsley or cilantro leaves

1. Preheat the oven to 400 degrees F.

2. Crumble the ground turkey in a large skillet and cook over medium-high heat until lightly browned. Drain off any fat, reduce the heat to medium, and add the onion, garlic, 1 cup of the chicken broth, tomato sauce, and cumin. Season with pepper and cook, stirring frequently, for 10 minutes. Stir in the rice until well combined. Remove the pan from the heat and let the mixture cool.

3. Place the pepper halves in a deep roasting pan. Fill the peppers with the turkey mixture and sprinkle with a little cheddar. Pour the remaining 1 cup of broth directly into the pan around the peppers. Bake for 20 minutes. Let the peppers cool slightly, sprinkle with the parsley or cilantro, and serve immediately.

Lemon-Scented Chicken Kebabs on Saffron Rice

SERVES 4

▶ *CALORIES PER SERVING* **490** // *SODIUM PER SERVING* **111MG**

This dish pays homage to the sophisticated cuisine of Iran, where simple, subtly spiced dishes are made with ingredients that delight the senses as well as power and balance the body. Protein, vitamin C, and iron-rich, this dish is lightly aromatic with saffron and lemon and low in sodium. Note that if you use wooden skewers for the kebabs, they should be soaked in water for at least 30 minutes before using.

2 skinless, boneless chicken breasts, cut into 1-inch cubes

½ cup freshly squeezed lemon juice

2 tablespoons lemon zest

2 tablespoons thyme leaves

⅛ teaspoon saffron powder

2–3 tablespoons extra-virgin olive oil, divided

1 cup basmati rice

1 pint cherry tomatoes

1. Put the chicken in a large sealable plastic bag and add the lemon juice, zest, and thyme. Shake the bag vigorously to coat. Let the chicken sit in the refrigerator for 1 hour, shaking the bag from time to time.

2. In a small bowl, soak the saffron powder in ½ cup boiling water. Heat 1–2 tablespoons of the oil (enough to coat the bottom of the pan) in a medium saucepan over medium-high heat. Add the rice and cook for about 5 minutes, stirring well to make sure the rice is evenly coated with oil. Add 1½ cups boiling water and the saffron water to the pan, cover, and cook for 20 minutes until the rice is tender and the liquid has been absorbed.

continued ▶

3. Meanwhile, thread the kebabs. Drain the chicken and pat dry with paper towels. Thread alternating pieces of chicken and tomatoes on metal or wooden skewers until each skewer is full.

4. Broil or grill the kebabs for about 5 minutes on each side, or until the chicken is cooked through and the tomatoes are bursting. Pile the rice on a large platter, lay the kebabs on top, and serve immediately.

Panko-Crusted Chicken Strips with Apricot Dipping Sauce

SERVES 4

▶ *CALORIES PER SERVING* **491** // *SODIUM PER SERVING* **435MG**

These chicken strips are made just for adults. They are coated with panko bread-crumbs and baked to a perfect crunch. An easy-to-make apricot sauce adds a touch of sophistication, elevating the dish above the mundane honey-mustard world where chicken strips usually reside.

1½ pounds skinless, boneless chicken breasts, cut lengthwise into 1-inch-wide strips
½ cup low-fat buttermilk
4 cups panko breadcrumbs
Freshly ground pepper
¼ cup apricot jam
3 tablespoons freshly squeezed lemon juice
2 teaspoons Dijon mustard

1. Preheat the oven to 400° F.

2. Put the chicken strips and buttermilk in a large bowl, stir to coat completely, and refrigerate for 1 hour.

3. Put the panko in a large shallow dish and season with pepper. Roll a piece of chicken in the panko until completely coated, and transfer it to a rimmed baking sheet. Repeat with the remaining chicken. Bake for 8 minutes, or until the chicken is crisp on the outside and cooked through. Let cool slightly.

4. In a small bowl, whisk together the jam, lemon juice, and mustard. Serve alongside the chicken strips.

Best Practices Roast Chicken

SERVES 6

▸ *CALORIES PER SERVING* **257** // *SODIUM PER SERVING* **104MG**

There are as many "foolproof" ways to roast a chicken as there are home cooks. Here, several of the best have been combined to provide you with the ultimate roast chicken. This is a great technique: Take a peek through the oven window to watch the heat transform the humble chicken.

1 (4-5-pound) roasting chicken
Juice of 1 orange
¼ cup extra-virgin olive oil
1 teaspoon ground cumin
2-4 small lemons
2-4 sprigs rosemary

1. Preheat the oven to 350° F.

2. Rinse the chicken under cold water and pat completely dry. Coat the chicken with the orange juice.

3. Whisk the oil and cumin in a small bowl. Pulling back the skin of the chicken wherever possible, pour a little of the oil mixture between the meat and skin. Work it in with your fingers.

4. Poke small holes in the lemons with a knife. Place loosely in the chicken cavity and tuck the rosemary in around them. Close the cavity by tying the legs or by using toothpicks to secure the skin flap.

5. Bake the chicken for 45 minutes. Without opening the oven door, increase the temperature to 450° F and cook for another 15 minutes, or until the internal temperature registers 165° F on an instant-read meat thermometer and the thigh juices run clear. Let the chicken rest for 20 minutes before carving.

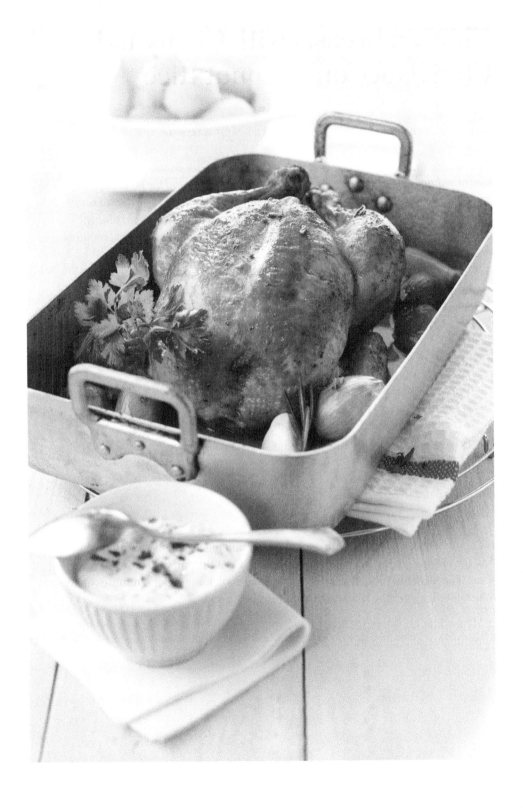

Chicken Breasts with Citrus and Chili Sauce on Coconut Rice

SERVES 4

▶ *CALORIES PER SERVING* **405** // *SODIUM PER SERVING* **112MG**

Low in sodium, this dish uses the vitamin C power of citrus and the potassium and magnesium in coconut to create a delicious dinner that is heart-healthy and simple to prepare. This recipe is perfect for a quick yet sophisticated weeknight dinner. The chicken preparation is simple and straightforward, and the sauce just requires deglazing.

Cooking spray

2 skinless, boneless chicken breasts, split in half

1 cup long-grain brown rice

2 cups coconut water

½ cup low-fat milk

1 teaspoon all-purpose flour

1 teaspoon cornstarch

½ cup freshly squeezed orange juice with pulp

3 tablespoons freshly squeezed lime juice

3-6 hot chili peppers (Thai bird, jalapeño, or habanero), halved, seeded, de-ribbed, and thinly sliced

Freshly ground pepper

1. Thinly coat a large skillet with cooking spray and place over medium-high heat. Add the chicken, cover, and cook for 4 minutes. Coat the pan with more cooking spray if needed, flip the chicken over, cover, and cook for another 4 minutes on the other side. Transfer the chicken to a plate and set aside.

2. Meanwhile, cook the rice according to package directions, using the coconut water instead of regular water for cooking.

3. In a small bowl, whisk together the milk, flour, and cornstarch and set aside.

4. Pour the orange juice into the skillet and place over high heat. Bring the juice to a boil, stirring constantly with a fork to scrape up any brown bits from the pan. Add the lime juice and chilies and cook for 3 minutes. Reduce the heat to medium and stir in the milk mixture, whisking until smooth and well incorporated. Return the chicken to the pan and cook for 3–5 minutes, or until the chicken is heated through. Serve the chicken and sauce over the coconut rice.

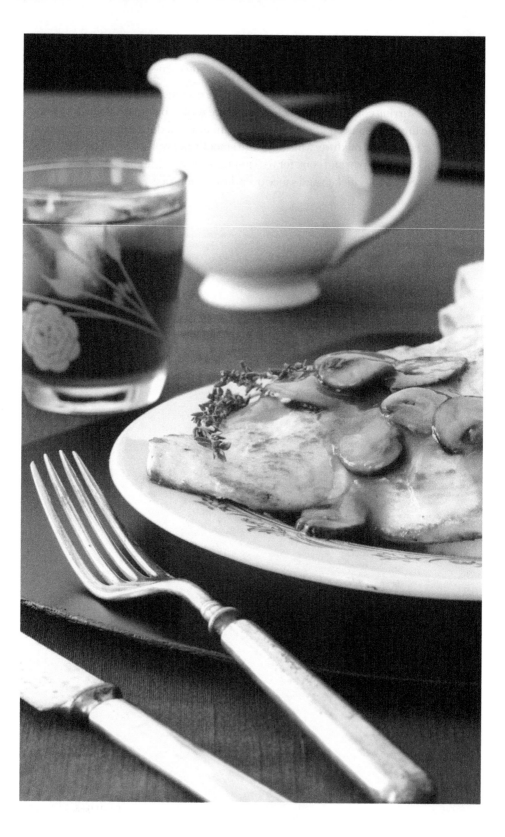

Chicken Breasts with Mushroom Sauce on Wild Rice

SERVES 4

▸ *CALORIES PER SERVING* **407** // *SODIUM PER SERVING* **114MG**

This simple preparation, cooking the chicken and deglazing the pan, is great for a quick weeknight dinner and provides niacin, folate, copper, zinc, and a host of other essential nutrients. Wild rice provides dietary fiber and a nutty, delicious base for the dish.

Cooking spray

2 skinless, boneless chicken breasts, split in half

1 cup wild rice

2 tablespoons extra-virgin olive oil

2 cups sliced assorted mushrooms, including white, crimini, and oyster

2 shallots, finely diced

2 teaspoons dried sage

½ cup low-sodium chicken or vegetable broth

½ cup chopped parsley

1. Thinly coat a large skillet with cooking spray and place over medium-high heat. Add the chicken, cover, and cook for 4 minutes. Coat the pan with more cooking spray if needed, flip the chicken over, cover, and cook on the other side for 4 minutes. Transfer the chicken to a plate and set aside.

2. Meanwhile, wash the rice under cold running water, rubbing the grains between your fingers. Put 3 cups water and the rice in a medium saucepan, bring to a boil, and cook over medium heat, covered, 45–60 minutes, or until tender.

3. Add the oil to the skillet and place over medium-high heat. Add the mushrooms, shallots, and sage, and cook, stirring frequently, until the mushrooms release their liquid, about 5 minutes. Add the broth and cook, stirring frequently to scrape any brown bits from the pan, for 5 minutes, or until the sauce thickens.

4. Return the chicken to the pan and cook for 3–5 minutes, or until the chicken is heated through. Remove the pan from the heat and sprinkle with the parsley. Serve the chicken and mushroom sauce over the wild rice.

Chicken Breasts with Mango-Rosemary Sauce on Brown Rice

SERVES 4

▶ *CALORIES PER SERVING* **381** // *SODIUM PER SERVING* **109MG**

Another healthy, quick chicken dish, this recipe pairs the startling flavor combination of mango and rosemary and provides the body with good amounts of vitamins A and C.

Cooking spray
2 skinless, boneless chicken breasts, split in half
1 cup long-grain brown rice
1 cup low-sodium chicken broth
1 cup mango juice
2 ripe mangos, peeled and coarsely chopped
Juice of 1 lime
2 tablespoons chopped rosemary leaves
Freshly ground pepper

1. Thinly coat a large skillet with cooking spray and place over medium-high heat. Add the chicken, cover, and cook for 4 minutes. Coat the pan with more cooking spray if needed, flip the chicken over, cover, and cook on the other side for 4 minutes. Transfer the chicken to a plate and set aside.

2. Meanwhile, cook the rice according to package directions.

3. Pour the chicken broth and mango juice into the skillet and place over medium-high heat. Bring the liquid to a boil, stirring constantly with a fork to scrape up any brown bits from the pan, and cook until the liquid is reduced by half. Add the chopped mango, lime juice, and rosemary, and stir well. Return the chicken to the pan and cook for 3–5 minutes, or until the chicken is heated through. Serve the chicken and sauce over the rice.

The Winemaker's Feast

SERVES 4

▶ *CALORIES PER SERVING* **445** // *SODIUM PER SERVING* **194MG**

Grapes are the star ingredient here and fresh pork sausage is a close second. The sausage must be fresh, or the sodium content is simply too high. Find it in the meat section, not where the precooked sausages are—that's the bad part of town, sodium-wise. This dish is also good with whole-wheat spaghetti.

2 pounds red seedless grapes, halved

2-3 tablespoons extra-virgin olive oil

4 sprigs rosemary, leaves chopped

½ teaspoon freshly ground pepper

4 fresh pork sausages

1 (12-ounce) package egg noodles

1. Preheat the oven to 350 degrees F.

2. Fill a shallow casserole or baking dish with the grapes. Add the oil, rosemary leaves, and pepper, and stir well to coat. Lay the sausages on top of the grapes.

3. Bake for 30–40 minutes, turning the sausages over halfway through the cooking. The sausages should be brown and look juicy, and the grapes should be soft and nearly liquefied. Transfer the sausages to a plate.

4. Cook the noodles according to the package directions, then drain.

5. Add the noodles to the casserole and toss well with the grape mixture. Divide the noodles among 4 plates and place a sausage on top of each. Serve immediately.

Grilled Pork Tenderloin with Garlic and Herbs

SERVES 6

▸ *CALORIES PER SERVING* **178** // *SODIUM PER SERVING* **48MG**

Pork tenderloin is always a showstopper when entertaining. Since it's so low in fat, stuff it full of herbs and garlic to flavor the meat as it cooks. And you'll have plenty of leftovers to tuck into sandwiches and to dress up salads.

1 (3-pound) pork tenderloin
2 tablespoons extra-virgin olive oil
4 garlic cloves, minced
2 tablespoons chopped thyme leaves
4 or 5 small sprigs rosemary

1. Preheat a grill to medium-high heat.

2. Make an incision about 1 inch deep along the entire length of the fatty side of the tenderloin. Rub the tenderloin with the oil, including inside the cut.

3. Pack the incision with the garlic, thyme, and rosemary, then pinch it shut. Grill the pork for 1 hour, turning it every 15 minutes, or until the internal temperature registers 145° F on an instant-read thermometer.

4. Let the tenderloin rest for 15 minutes before slicing and serving.

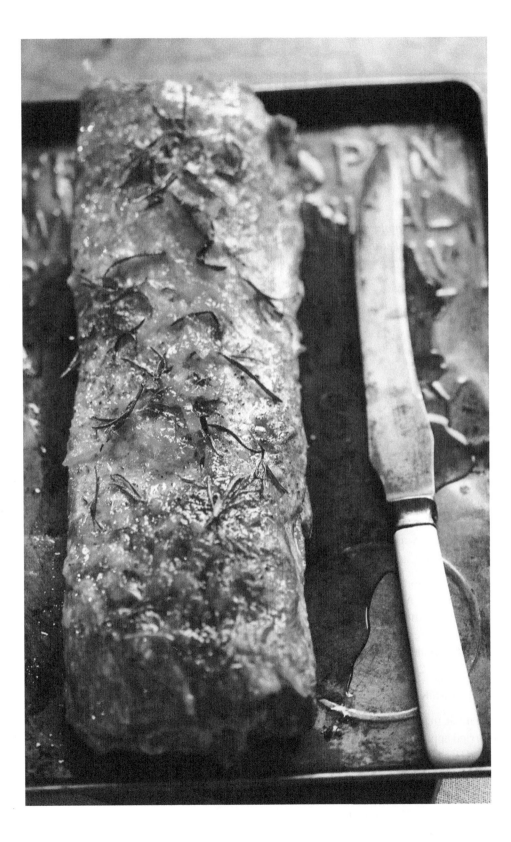

Boneless Pork Chops with Curried Apples

SERVES 4

▸ *CALORIES PER SERVING* **583** // *SODIUM PER SERVING* **102MG**

Pork and apples make a handsome pair and a warming winter meal. Try throwing a handful of dried cranberries, currants, raisins, or toasted pecans into the apple mixture just before serving, if desired. For variety, serve over rice, quinoa, bulgur, or kasha.

2 tablespoons extra-virgin olive oil

4 lean boneless pork chops

1 large onion, coarsely chopped

4 medium McIntosh or Winesap apples, peeled, cored, and thinly sliced

1 cup apple juice

2–3 tablespoons curry powder

Freshly ground pepper

1 (12-ounce) package egg noodles

1. Heat the oil in a large heavy-bottomed skillet or cast-iron pan over medium-high heat. Add the pork chops and brown on one side for 1–2 minutes; then flip the chops and brown on the other side for 1–2 minutes. Transfer the pork to a plate and set aside.

2. Add the onion to the skillet. Reduce the heat to low and cook until just softened, 8–10 minutes. Add the apples, apple juice, and curry, and mix thoroughly. Season with pepper. Increase the heat to maintain a gentle simmer for 10 minutes. Return the pork to the skillet, cover with the apples, and cook for 10 minutes. (If the sauce is too thin, continue to cook on high for 1–2 minutes to reduce it; if the sauce is too thick, add 1–2 tablespoons water.)

3. Meanwhile, cook the noodles according to the package directions. Drain.

4. Divide the noodles among 4 plates. Place a pork chop on top and cover with the curried apples. Serve immediately.

Scottish Meatloaf

SERVES 4

▸*CALORIES PER SERVING* **400** // *SODIUM PER SERVING* **175MG**

Home cooks know that a good meatloaf recipe is worth its weight in gold. Here you can stuff a meatloaf with hard-boiled eggs as the Scots do, or try a layer of sautéed mushrooms and low-sodium cheese.

4 large eggs
¼ cup low-fat milk
1 cup old-fashioned oats
1½ pounds lean ground beef
¼ cup chopped parsley leaves
1 tablespoon dried sage
1 teaspoon reduced-sodium Worcestershire sauce
Freshly ground pepper
2 tablespoons extra-virgin olive oil
2 large onions, coarsely chopped

1. Preheat the oven to 400° F.

2. Boil 3 of the eggs for 7 minutes. Place under cold running water to cool. When cool enough to handle, peel and set aside.

3. In a large bowl, beat the remaining egg and milk with a whisk. Add the oats, stir well, and let sit for at least 5 minutes, or until the oats absorb the liquid and soften. Stir in the beef, parsley, sage, and Worcestershire sauce, and season with pepper.

4. Heat the oil in a medium skillet over medium-high heat. Add the onions, reduce the heat to medium, and cook until translucent, about 10 minutes. Scrape the onions and oil into the meat mixture. Work the mixture together with a wooden spoon or clean hands until all of the ingredients are thoroughly combined.

5. Spread half of the beef mixture in the bottom of a loaf pan. Lay the hard-boiled eggs end to end down the center of the mixture. Top the eggs with the remaining mixture and smooth the top. Bake the meatloaf for 1 hour. Let it rest for 5 minutes before slicing and serve with a drizzle of pan juices over each slice.

Argentinean-Style Flank Steak

SERVES 4

▶ *CALORIES PER SERVING* **390** // *SODIUM PER SERVING* **387MG**

For a meat lover, this is one of the easiest, most delicious ways to prepare steak. In Argentina, you can pull off the road in the countryside for some asado, or grilled meats marinated in lemon and salt, that melts in the mouth. Here, we use a tiny amount of sea salt, which has less sodium than iodized salt and will tenderize the meat nicely. Slice the flank steak against the grain and serve atop a bed of Massaged Kale Salad (page 138) for a sophisticated dish worthy of a five-star restaurant.

1–1½ pounds flank steak

Juice of 1 lemon

½ teaspoon sea salt

1 tablespoon extra-virgin olive oil or canola oil

1. Rinse the flank steak under cold running water and pat dry with paper towels. Place the meat in a shallow dish and rub all sides with the lemon juice. Spread ¼ teaspoon sea salt on each side and let the steak sit at room temperature for 2–4 hours. Remove the steak and pat dry with paper towels.

2. Heat the oil over medium-high heat in a large skillet that can hold the steak comfortably. For a rare steak, sear for about 3 minutes per side. Add 1 minute or more per side for a more well-done steak.

3. Transfer the steak to a cutting board and let it rest for 10 minutes. Do not skip this step! Cut the steak against the grain into long, thin slices. Serve over kale or other vegetables with the pan juices drizzled on top.

Pot Roast with Sweet Potatoes, Peas, and Onions

SERVES 6

▶ *CALORIES PER SERVING* **615** // *SODIUM PER SERVING* **202MG**

Sweet potatoes are a fabulous replacement for the white ones that usually grace the monolithic cuts of beef. Here, the pot roast cooks in a large amount of liquid, almost creating a stew. Serve the melt-in-your-mouth beef in a bowl with the juices and vegetables.

1 (3– 4-pound) beef pot roast
Freshly ground pepper
1 tablespoon extra-virgin olive oil
1 (14.5-ounce) can low-sodium beef broth
1 cup red wine
1 large onion, diced
1 carrot, peeled and cut into 1-inch coins
2 garlic cloves, chopped
1 cinnamon stick
3 large sweet potatoes, peeled and diced into 1-inch cubes
1 (10-ounce) package frozen peas
Juice of ½ lemon
½ cup chopped parsley leaves
¼ cup chopped rosemary and/or thyme leaves

1. Rinse the roast under cold running water and pat dry with paper towels. Roll the roast in pepper on all sides.

2. Heat the oil in a large stockpot over medium-high heat. Cook the roast, turning every few minutes, until browned on all sides, about 8 minutes. Remove the pot from the heat.

3. Pour the broth and wine over the beef. Add the onion, carrot, garlic, and cinnamon stick to the pot and enough water to cover the meat. Bring to a boil over high

continued ▶

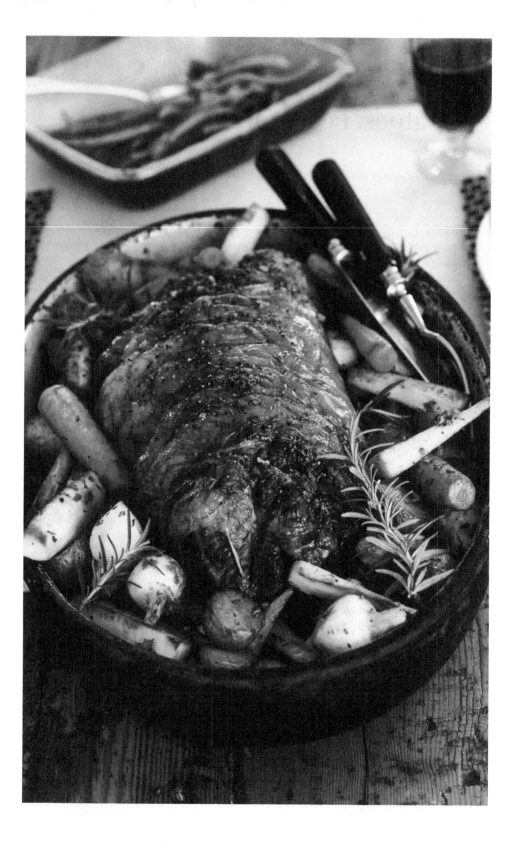

heat, then reduce the heat to medium and simmer for 3 hours, adding more water or broth as needed.

4. Add the sweet potatoes and simmer for 30 minutes. Add the peas and cook for 10 minutes.

5. Remove the pan from the heat. Stir in the lemon juice, parsley, and rosemary. Transfer the roast to a deep platter and spoon the vegetables and liquid around it. Serve immediately.

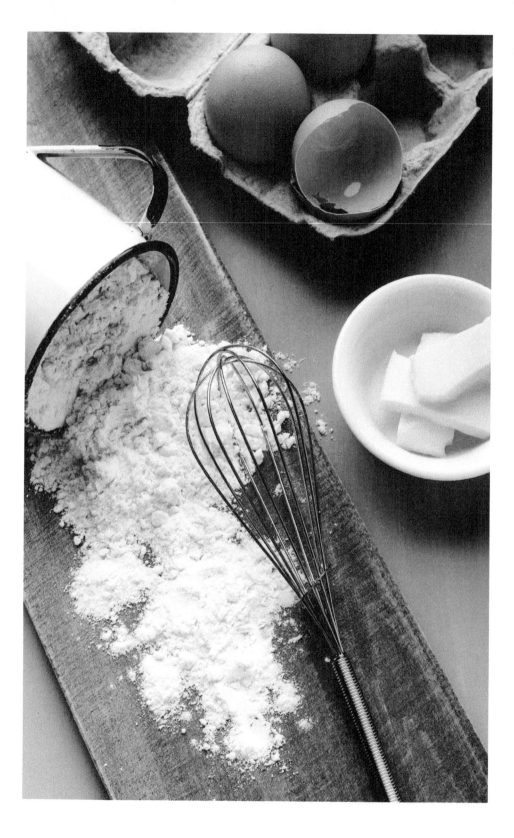

CHAPTER SIXTEEN

DASH Desserts

- ▶ Watermelon Ice
- ▶ Cantaloupe Granita
- ▶ Herbed Grapefruit Sorbet
- ▶ Lemonade Ice Pops
- ▶ Soy Milk Shakes
- ▶ Cherries, Almonds, and Cheese
- ▶ Tea and Jam Platter
- ▶ Fruit Sauce for Sundaes
- ▶ Rhubarb Compote
- ▶ Vanilla and Lemon Berry Parfaits
- ▶ Balsamic Berries
- ▶ Coconut Soup
- ▶ Chocolate Pudding
- ▶ Frozen Chocolate Cannoli Sandwiches
- ▶ Candied Pecans
- ▶ Dark Chocolate Almond Clusters

- ▶ Figs Baked with Goat Cheese and Honey
- ▶ Fig Cookies
- ▶ Heart-Healing Chocolate Chip Cookies
- ▶ Meringue Kisses
- ▶ Dark Chocolate–Covered Fruits
- ▶ Pears Poached in Orange Juice and Red Wine
- ▶ Grilled Peaches
- ▶ Clafouti
- ▶ Berry Apple Cobbler
- ▶ Lighten Up Brownies
- ▶ Berries in Meringue
- ▶ Homemade Chocolate-Hazelnut Spread
- ▶ Basic Cheesecake
- ▶ Chocolate Olive Oil Cake

Watermelon Ice

SERVES 6

▶ *CALORIES PER SERVING* **229** // *SODIUM PER SERVING* **18MG**

A tasty, low-calorie fruit, watermelon is full of vitamins A and C and potassium, with virtually no sodium. A carefree dessert, it's like summertime for your mouth.

½ medium seedless watermelon
1 (15.25-ounce) can crushed pineapple with liquid
1 (6-ounce) can frozen lemonade
⅓ cup sugar
1 tablespoon freshly squeezed lemon juice

1. Scoop the watermelon flesh into the bowl of a food processor and process until you have 8 cups. Strain the juice through a fine-mesh sieve to remove the pulp. Discard the pulp. Transfer the juice to a large bowl.

2. Add the pineapple and juice, lemonade, sugar, and lemon juice to the bowl. Stir with a whisk until the sugar dissolves.

3. Pour the watermelon mixture into an 8 × 13-inch metal pan or tray. Freeze until solid. Using a sharp knife, break the frozen mixture into chunks. Transfer the chunks to a food processor or blender and process until smooth. Serve immediately.

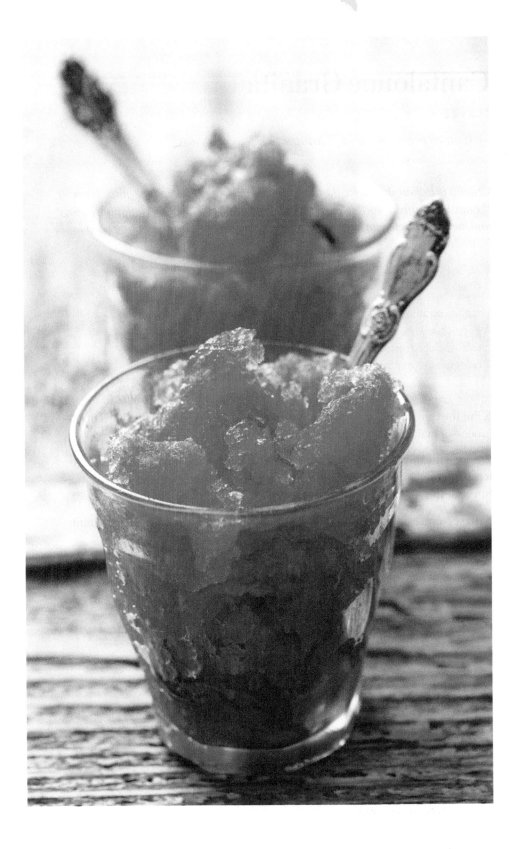

Cantaloupe Granita

SERVES 4

▶ *CALORIES PER SERVING* **89** // *SODIUM PER SERVING* **19MG**

Granita is Italian shaved ice that when served in a small champagne glass, is one of the most beautiful, colorful, and simplest desserts on earth. The technique is so easy and the result so elegant, no one will ever suspect there's a healthy eating agenda behind it.

1 large cantaloupe, seeded and cut into large chunks
1 cup ice cubes
¼ cup sugar
2 tablespoons freshly squeezed lemon juice
2 tablespoons minced fresh mint, plus whole mint leaves for garnish

1. Put the cantaloupe, ice, sugar, lemon juice, and minced mint in the bowl of a food processor or a blender and process until smooth.

2. Spoon the mixture into a shallow baking dish or freezer tray and freeze for at least 40 minutes, preferably 2–3 hours. Occasionally run a fork through the mixture as it freezes to form more ice crystals.

3. To serve, use a fork to skim layers of granita into 4 glasses. Garnish with mint leaves and serve immediately.

Herbed Grapefruit Sorbet

SERVES 4

▶ *CALORIES PER SERVING* **266** // *SODIUM PER SERVING* **1MG**

You'll need an ice-cream maker to make this sorbet. But don't worry, if you don't have one, simply turn this into grapefruit granita by following the instructions on the previous page. Pairing herbs with fruit is a unique and delicious detail in this sorbet.

3 cups freshly squeezed pink grapefruit juice, divided
¾ cup sugar
2 tablespoons shredded basil leaves or chopped thyme or mint

1. Combine ½ cup of the grapefruit juice and the sugar in a medium saucepan and bring to a boil over medium-high heat and cook, stirring frequently, until the sugar dissolves. Transfer the sugar mixture to a medium bowl, cover, and refrigerate until completely cool.

2. Combine the sugar mixture with the remaining 2½ cups grapefruit juice. Pour into an ice-cream maker and process according to the manufacturer's directions.

3. Scoop the sorbet into tall glasses and sprinkle with the basil. Serve with a chilled teaspoon.

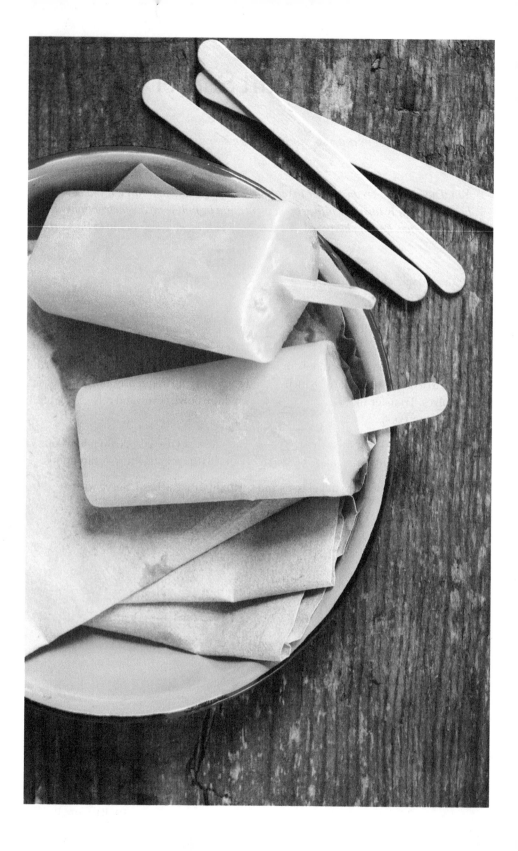

Lemonade Ice Pops

SERVES 4

▶ *CALORIES PER SERVING* **241** // *SODIUM PER SERVING* **2MG**

Make the ten-dollar investment in ice pop molds and have access to a lifetime of really good icy treats in your freezer. Any fresh fruit juice makes a magnificent ice pop, and you can even freeze juices in layers, creating striped ice pops with endless flavor combinations. Sure, these are definitely kid-pleasers, but hand one to someone who has been working hard and watch a smile spread across their face.

1⅓ cup freshly squeezed lemon juice
⅔ cup sugar
⅔ cup freshly squeezed orange juice
1 tablespoon lemon zest
½ teaspoon orange extract

1. Combine the lemon juice, 1 cup water, and sugar in a medium saucepan over high heat. Boil vigorously for 30 seconds to dissolve the sugar; then transfer to a large bowl. Add the orange juice, lemon zest, and orange extract, and mix thoroughly. Let cool for 15 minutes, then cover and refrigerate for at least 1 hour.

2. Pour the mixture into ice pop molds and freeze for at least 4 hours, or until the ice pops are frozen solid.

Soy Milk Shakes

SERVES 2

▶ *CALORIES PER SERVING* **285** *// SODIUM PER SERVING* **200MG**

Americans love milk shakes almost as much as they love soda, but the traditional ice cream and milk combination is packed with empty calories and not so great for the heart. This sweet, cold treat is much less detrimental to your health.

1⅓ cups vanilla or chocolate soy milk
3 cups fat-free vanilla or chocolate frozen yogurt
1 teaspoon freshly squeezed lemon juice

1. Put all of the ingredients in a blender and process until smooth. Pour into glasses and serve immediately.

Cherries, Almonds, and Cheese

SERVES 4

▶ *CALORIES PER SERVING* **161** // *SODIUM PER SERVING* **75MG**

This recipe is about the power of a few exceptional and harmonious ingredients. Toast the almonds in a dry skillet over medium heat for a few minutes until they brown slightly and their aroma fills your kitchen.

4 cups frozen pitted cherries
½ cup part-skim ricotta cheese
¼ cup slivered almonds, toasted
1 teaspoon ground cinnamon, for garnish

1. Heat the cherries in a glass dish in the microwave on high for 2–3 minutes, or until heated through. Alternatively, heat the cherries in a medium saucepan over medium heat until hot.

2. In bowls or stemmed glasses, spoon the cherries into the bottom, top with a dollop of ricotta, sprinkle with the almonds, and dust with a little cinnamon. Serve immediately.

Tea and Jam Platter

SERVES 6

▶ *CALORIES PER SERVING* **40** // *SODIUM PER SERVING* **0MG**

This dessert combines two cultures: black tea sweetened with jam (Russian) and served with cookies (American). It's an elegant combination that is perfectly suited for conversation in the living room. No one will mind drinking tea around the coffee table!

¼ cup blackberry jam
¼ cup strawberry jam
¼ cup raspberry jam
¼ cup orange marmalade
Assorted black teas
12 assorted cookies (pages 297, 298, and 301)

1. Place each jam in a small bowl. Fill a large teapot with hot (not boiling) water. Add 6 teabags or ¼ cup of loose tea. Let steep for 2 minutes, and then remove.

2. Serve the tea in small cups with teaspoons for stirring in the jam. Serve an assortment of cookies piled high on a platter.

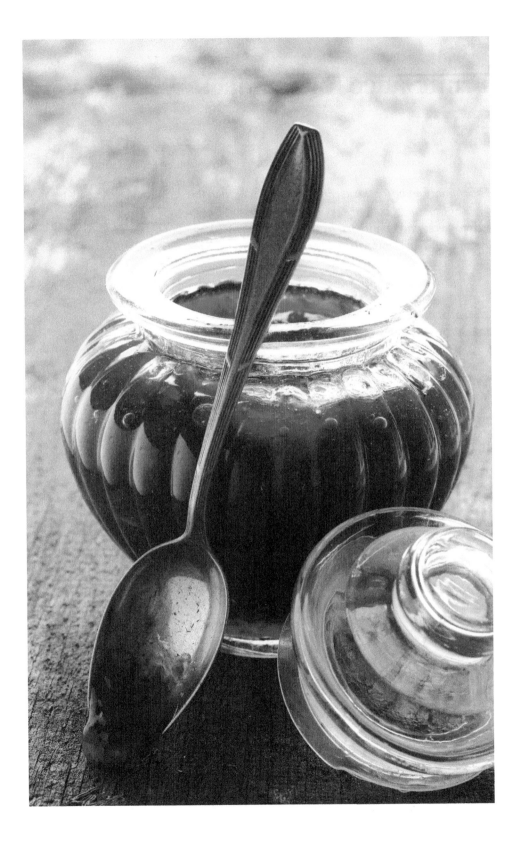

Fruit Sauce for Sundaes

SERVES 6

▶ *CALORIES PER SERVING* **98** // *SODIUM PER SERVING* **2MG**

The culinary name for thick fruit sauce is "coulis," and this recipe makes three. Place a piece of chocolate cake in a pool of raspberry sauce, or mix it with low-fat whipped cream cheese and sandwich it between graham crackers, or put a few small scoops of frozen yogurt in a bowl with a different sauce on each scoop for a beautiful sundae.

1 pint fresh or 1 (12-ounce) package frozen strawberries, blueberries, or raspberries
2 tablespoons sugar
2 tablespoons freshly squeezed lemon juice

1. To make the strawberry or blueberry sauce, combine all the ingredients in a blender or food processor, process until smooth, and serve at room temperature or chilled. To make the raspberry sauce, combine all of the ingredients in a blender or food processor and process until smooth. Strain the raspberry sauce through a fine-mesh sieve and discard the seeds. Serve the sauce at room temperature or chilled.

Rhubarb Compote

SERVES 4

▸ *CALORIES PER SERVING* **244** // *SODIUM PER SERVING* **1MG**

Rhubarb is one of the first fruits of summer. Its flavor is tart and bracing and can be a bit of an acquired taste. Once you learn to love rhubarb, though, there is no turning back.

4 cups rhubarb, cut in ½-inch pieces
½ cup sugar

1. Combine the rhubarb and sugar in a large saucepan and let it sit until the rhubarb begins releasing its juices, about 10 minutes.

2. Place the saucepan over high heat and stir constantly while it comes to a boil. Reduce the heat to maintain a simmer, cover, and cook for 10–12 minutes, or until the rhubarb is tender. Remove the pan from the heat and let the rhubarb cool without stirring. Refrigerate for at least 2 hours before serving.

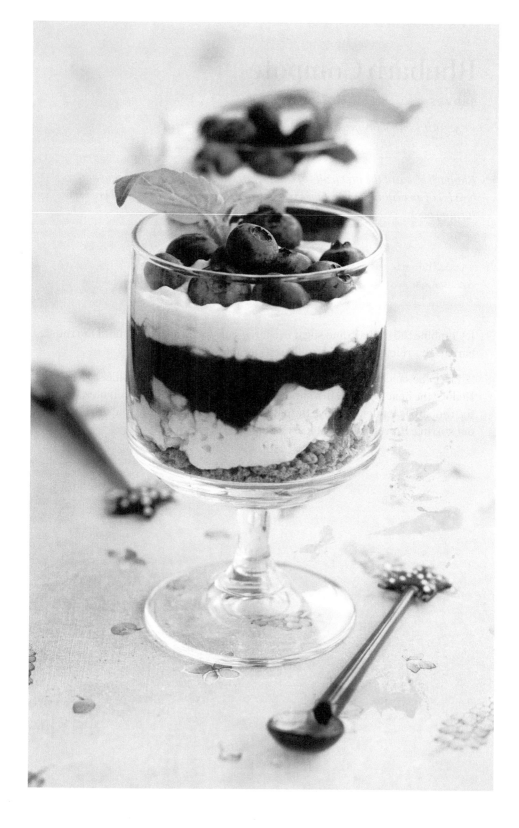

Vanilla and Lemon Berry Parfaits

SERVES 4

▶ *CALORIES PER SERVING* **240** // *SODIUM PER SERVING* **193MG**

Nonfat yogurt is pumped full of lemon and vanilla to provide creamy layers between fresh berries. Arrange the parfaits in water tumblers for a casual meal and in champagne or wine glasses for fancier fare.

2 cups nonfat vanilla yogurt
1 (3.4-ounce) box fat-free vanilla instant pudding
3 tablespoons lemon curd, such as Dickinson's
1 teaspoon vanilla extract
1 tablespoon honey
Zest and juice of 1 lemon
4 cups fresh mixed berries, such as blueberries, raspberries,
    strawberries, or blackberries
Mint leaves, for garnish

1. Combine the yogurt, instant pudding, lemon curd, and vanilla, and mix well.

2. Whisk together the honey and lemon zest and juice in a large bowl. Add the berries and stir gently with a spatula until they are well coated.

3. Spoon a 2-inch layer of the yogurt mixture into the bottom of a glass. Cover with a 2-inch layer of berries. Continue layering the yogurt and berries until the glass is full. Repeat with the remaining 3 glasses. Refrigerate the parfaits for at least 1 hour. Garnish with mint leaves before serving.

Balsamic Berries

SERVES 4

▶ *CALORIES PER SERVING* **76** // *SODIUM PER SERVING* **10MG**

Simple and sophisticated, fruit mixed with balsamic vinegar never fails to impress your foodie friends. It is a complex, delicious dessert that will please all.

1 cup sliced strawberries
1 cup blueberries
1 cup raspberries
¼ cup balsamic vinegar
2 tablespoons brown sugar
1 teaspoon vanilla extract
¼ cup nonfat vanilla yogurt
Shredded basil leaves, for garnish

1. In a large bowl, combine the strawberries, blueberries, and raspberries, and mix well.

2. In a small bowl, whisk together the vinegar, brown sugar, and vanilla. Pour the mixture over the fruit. Cover the bowl with plastic wrap and let it sit at room temperature for 1–2 hours, stirring every 15 minutes, to allow the flavors to meld.

3. Transfer the bowl to the refrigerator and chill for 1 hour before serving. Spoon the fruit into martini glasses, top with a dollop of the yogurt, and sprinkle with basil.

Coconut Soup

SERVES 4

▸ *CALORIES PER SERVING* **267** // *SODIUM PER SERVING* **169MG**

If you love Almond Joy or Mounds candy bars, this is the desert for you. Coconut milk is poured over chocolate and almonds for a low-sodium candy bar in a glass. Coconut provides lauric acid, which increases good cholesterol in the body as well as copper, calcium, manganese, magnesium, and zinc. Coconuts are probably the reason why islanders are so happy all the time.

1½ cups coconut milk

3 tablespoons palm, raw, or brown sugar

2 to 2½ cups coconut water

Zest of 1 lime

½ cup nonfat vanilla yogurt

½ cup dark chocolate chips

¼ cup unsweetened shredded coconut, toasted

¼ cup slivered almonds, toasted

1. In a large bowl, whisk the coconut milk and sugar together until the sugar dissolves. Stir in the coconut water until the soup reaches the desired thickness; then add the lime zest and stir well. Refrigerate the soup for at least 1 hour, or until the soup is very cold.

2. Spoon 2 tablespoons of the yogurt into a dessert bowl or cocktail glass, sprinkle with chocolate chips and shredded coconut, and pour the coconut soup around it. Garnish with almonds and serve immediately.

Chocolate Pudding

SERVES 6

▶ *CALORIES PER SERVING* **229** // *SODIUM PER SERVING* **54MG**

Avocado provides a match for the rich, creamy texture of milk fat. You must chill this pudding very well or you will taste a hint of avocado through the chocolate. Serve this in teacups or small elegant bowls at the end of a fancy meal, or simply spoon it into small paper cups and pair it with a good movie.

2 Hass avocados, cut into chunks

1 banana, cut into chunks

1 cup unsweetened almond milk

¼ cup unsweetened cocoa powder

2 tablespoons maple syrup

1 teaspoon vanilla extract

½ teaspoon ground cinnamon

1. Put all the ingredients in a blender or food processor and process until completely smooth. Transfer to a bowl, cover, and refrigerate for at least 4 hours. The pudding should be served very cold.

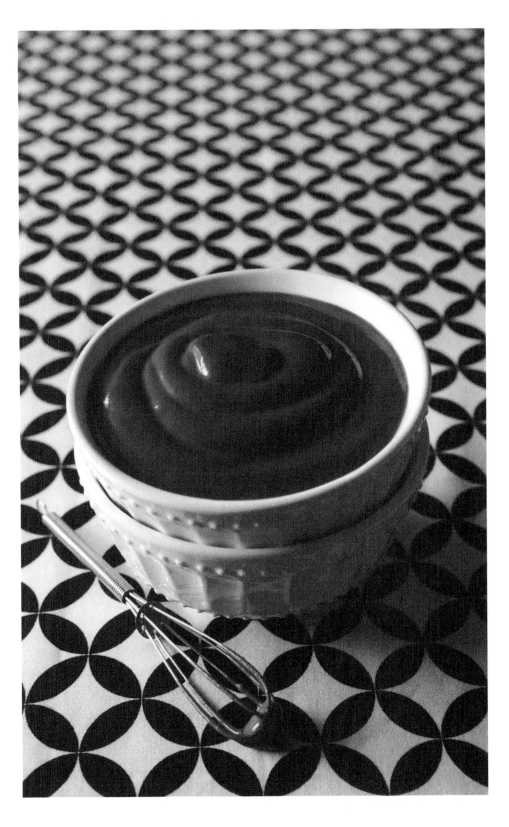

Frozen Chocolate Cannoli Sandwiches

SERVES 6, MAKES 1 DOZEN SANDWICHES

▶ *CALORIES PER SERVING* **279** // *SODIUM PER SERVING* **235MG**

A true cannoli is Italian pastry dough rolled into a tube, deep fried, and filled with sweetened ricotta and chocolate bits. For the DASH diet, we'll skip the deep-fried part and deliver the flavors of cannoli without the extra fat.

1 cup part-skim ricotta
2 tablespoons all-fruit apricot or orange marmalade
1 tablespoon sugar
1 teaspoon lemon zest
2 tablespoons mini chocolate chips
1 (10-ounce) box chocolate graham crackers

1. In a large bowl, combine the ricotta, marmalade, sugar, and lemon zest and beat with an electric mixer until thoroughly incorporated and light in texture. Fold in the chocolate chips.

2. Spread 2 tablespoons of the ricotta mixture on a graham cracker square and top with a second square, pressing down slightly to even out the filling. Repeat until all the ricotta is used.

3. Wrap each sandwich in waxed paper and freeze for 4–8 hours before serving.

Candied Pecans

SERVES 2

▸ *CALORIES PER SERVING* **167** // *SODIUM PER SERVING* **0MG**

Snacking, garnishing, and embellishing—that's what these sweet pecans are for. Choose big, meaty pecan halves to showcase the flavor. Put them on your cookie tray or toss them in a salad of arugula, goat cheese, and fresh strawberries.

Cooking spray
¾ cup sugar
Pinch of cream of tartar
1 cup pecan halves

1. Thinly coat a rimmed baking sheet with cooking spray.

2. In a medium saucepan, combine the sugar, ¼ cup water, and cream of tartar, and place over medium-low heat until the sugar dissolves. Increase the heat to medium-high and boil until the syrup is thick and a dark amber color, about 7 minutes. Watch it carefully so it doesn't burn. Remove the pan from heat and immediately stir in the pecans.

3. Spread the pecans on the baking sheet, separating them so they aren't touching. Leave a little bit of the caramel coating attached to each nut. Cool completely and store for up to 1 week in an airtight container.

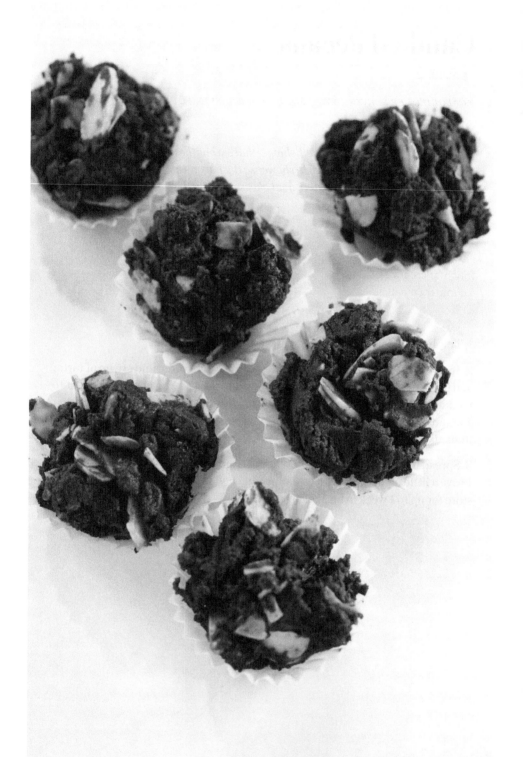

Dark Chocolate Almond Clusters

SERVES 4, 1 DOZEN CLUSTERS

▶ *CALORIES PER SERVING* **275** // *SODIUM PER SERVING* **17MG**

After you make these clusters successfully, try cashews and coconut, peanuts and crushed banana chips, hazelnuts and currants, or any other combination that strikes your fancy. If you refrigerate the clusters immediately, you do not have to temper the chocolate. If they must sit out at room temperature to cool, temper the chocolate according to the instructions on page 157 or the chocolate will "bloom" with white streaks.

1 cup almonds
5 ounces dark or bittersweet chocolate, chopped

1. Preheat the oven to 350° F.

2. Spread the almonds on a rimmed baking sheet and toast for 8 to 10 minutes, watching then carefully so they don't burn. Remove from the oven and let cool for several minutes. When the almonds are cool enough to handle, chop them roughly.

3. Bring water to a boil in the bottom of a double boiler. Put the chocolate in the top of the double boiler. Stir frequently until the chocolate melts.

4. Add the almond pieces to the chocolate and stir, coating the nuts well. Using a tablespoon, transfer a big cluster onto waxed paper. Repeat to make about 12 clusters, leaving a little space between each one. Refrigerate immediately for at least 1 hour before serving.

Figs Baked with Goat Cheese and Honey

SERVES 4

▶ *CALORIES PER SERVING* **331** // *SODIUM PER SERVING* **104MG**

This recipe tastes like something that would have been served in antiquity. Good things can last. Figs help the heart with lots of potassium and the waistline with lots of fiber. Walnuts are full of omega-3, a good fat for the human heart and brain.

4 large fresh figs, halved

4 ounces goat cheese

4 tablespoons honey

Freshly ground pepper

¼ cup walnut pieces

1. Preheat the oven to 350° F.

2. Arrange the figs cut side up on a rimmed baking sheet or shallow roasting pan.

3. Spoon ½ tablespoon of the goat cheese on each fig half, then drizzle with ½ tablespoon of the honey. Bake for 5–8 minutes, or just until the cheese has softened.

4. Arrange 2 fig halves on each dessert plate, topping them with another drizzle of honey, if desired. Season the figs lightly with pepper and scatter with walnuts. Serve immediately.

Fig Cookies

SERVES 8, MAKES 2 DOZEN COOKIES

▶ *CALORIES PER SERVING* **333** // *SODIUM PER SERVING* **143MG**

In the quest to avoid white flour, this ingenious recipe uses ground pecans and egg whites to give this cookie structure. Serve them with tea and jam (see page 282) or just with a glass of milk.

Cooking spray
¾ cup finely chopped Black Mission figs
2 tablespoons granulated sugar
1 cup chopped pecans
½ teaspoon ground cinnamon
1 tablespoon grated lemon zest
2 large egg whites
½ teaspoon cream of tartar
Pinch of salt
1½ cups confectioners' sugar

1. Preheat the oven to 300° F. Thinly coat 2 baking sheets with cooking spray.

2. Combine the figs and granulated sugar in a small bowl and set aside to let the flavors meld.

3. Add the pecans and cinnamon to the bowl of a food processor and process until the nuts are finely chopped. Add the lemon zest and continue to process until the mixture resembles coarse flour.

4. Combine the egg whites with the cream of tartar and salt in a large bowl. Beat with an electric mixer on high until the egg whites begin to form soft peaks when you raise the beaters. Gradually add the confectioners' sugar, beating after each addition, until all of the sugar is incorporated and the mixture is shiny and smooth.

5. Gently fold the pecan flour into the egg whites until completely incorporated. Gently fold in the figs with sugar.

6. Spoon large tablespoonfuls of the batter onto the baking sheets, leaving 1 inch between each cookie. Bake for 20 minutes. Let cool before serving.

Heart-Healing Chocolate Chip Cookies

SERVES 8, MAKES 2 DOZEN COOKIES

▶ *CALORIES PER SERVING* **604** // *SODIUM PER SERVING* **584MG**

Anyone who has ever bitten into a chocolate chip cookie understands immediately that it's a kind of medicine, a healer of hearts, a giver of comfort. This recipe includes healthy alternatives like oat flour standing in for all-purpose flour and rolled oats— the circulatory system's steadfast guardian—keeping the fiber factor high. Your veins, valves, and ventricles will thank you.

Cooking spray

2 cups walnuts

3 tablespoons canola oil

¾ cup brown sugar

2 teaspoons vanilla extract

1½ cups oat flour

1 teaspoon baking soda

½ teaspoon ground cinnamon

½ teaspoon ground nutmeg

Pinch of salt

2 cups rolled oats

1 (12-ounce) package dark or bittersweet chocolate chips

1. Preheat the oven to 350° F. Thinly coat 2 baking sheets with cooking spray.

2. In the bowl of a food processor, process the walnuts into fine flour. Add the oil and process for 2–3 minutes. The mixture should resemble natural nut butter. Leave the mixture in the food processor.

3. In a medium saucepan over medium-high heat, whisk together ½ cup water, the brown sugar, and vanilla, and stir constantly as it comes to a boil. Remove the pan from the heat. Let the mixture cool slightly before adding to the food processor with the nut mixture. Pulse a few times to incorporate.

continued ▶

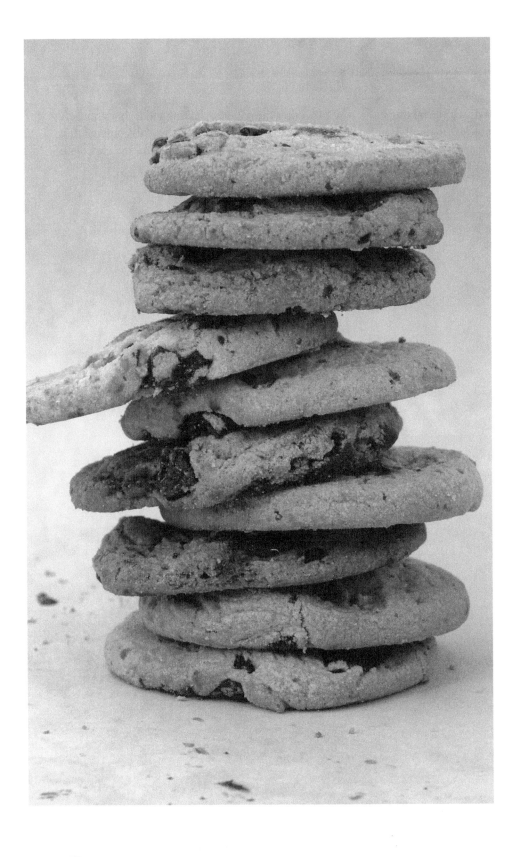

4. In a large mixing bowl, whisk together the oat flour, baking soda, cinnamon, nutmeg, and salt. Pour the nut mixture into the bowl and stir well to combine thoroughly. Let the dough rest for 10 minutes before stirring in the oats and chocolate.

5. Drop tablespoonfuls of the dough on the baking sheets, leaving 1 inch between each cookie, and bake for 8–10 minutes. Let cool before serving.

Meringue Kisses

SERVES 8, MAKES 2 DOZEN KISSES

▸ *CALORIES PER SERVING* **152** // *SODIUM PER SERVING* **472MG**

More like candy than cookies, these little gems will look beautiful on your cookie platter. Divide the batter and have a little fun with food coloring, turning the kisses different colors.

Cooking spray (optional)
4 large egg whites
½ teaspoon cream of tartar
Pinch of salt
1 teaspoon vanilla extract
1 cup sugar
8 ounces semisweet mini chocolate chips

1. Preheat the oven to 375° F. Thinly coat 2 baking sheets with cooking spray or line with parchment paper.

2. In a large bowl, combine the egg whites, cream of tartar, and salt. Beat with an electric mixer until peaks begin to form. Add the vanilla and 1 tablespoon of the sugar, and beat well. Continue beating and add the remaining sugar 1 tablespoon at a time. The whites will be glossy and thick. Gently fold in the chocolate chips.

3. If you have a pastry bag, fill it with the meringue and pipe it out into shapes. Alternately, drop the batter onto the baking sheets by the teaspoonful, forming a nice curl on the top.

4. Put the pans in the oven and immediately turn off the heat. Leave the cookies in the oven for 5 hours. Remove the cookies from the oven and serve.

Dark Chocolate–Covered Fruits

SERVES 6

▶ *CALORIES PER SERVING* **311** // *SODIUM PER SERVING* **1MG**

This recipe uses a simple technique—tempering chocolate—that creates elegant desserts. When tempering, chocolate is melted to a specific temperature, removed from the heat until the temperature drops, and then is returned to the heat for one last rise that creates shiny, streak-free chocolate worthy of professionals. A candy thermometer is a must for this recipe. Remember, chocolate hates water, so don't dip any fruit unless it's completely dry. Pile the coated fruit on a platter with unsalted pistachios and cashews for a show-stopping end to a meal.

1-pound block dark baking chocolate
1 quart large strawberries, rinsed and dried thoroughly
4 large oranges, peeled, sectioned, with pith and membrane removed
1 large grapefruit, peeled, sectioned, with pith and membrane removed
1 small pineapple, cut into bite-sized chunks

1. With a large sharp knife, chop the chocolate block at the edges, creating piles of shavings. Keep rotating the block and shaving off the corners until all of the chocolate has been shaved.

2. Bring water to a boil in the lower part of a double boiler. Put three-quarters of the chocolate shavings in the top and place a candy thermometer in the pan. Heat over the simmering water until the chocolate temperature hits 115° F.

3. Remove the top pan from the heat immediately and let the chocolate temperature drop to 84° F, stirring occasionally.

4. Return the top pan to the double boiler, add the remaining chocolate shavings, and stir constantly until the chocolate temperature rises to 89° F. Remove the pan from the heat and stir the chocolate as it cools.

5. Dip the fruit into the chocolate and place on waxed paper so the chocolate can harden. Store in an airtight container in the refrigerator until ready to serve. Arrange on a platter and serve.

Pears Poached in Orange Juice and Red Wine

SERVES 4

▶ *CALORIES PER SERVING* **206** // *SODIUM PER SERVING* **24MG**

Pears poached in red wine turn a beautiful color as the alcohol evaporates, creating a supremely elegant dessert. Use a good red wine for this. It makes a big difference to the dish's flavor.

2 cups red wine
Juice of 1 orange
¼ cup sugar
2 cinnamon sticks
1 tablespoon whole cloves
4 firm ripe pears
¼ cup low-fat vanilla yogurt
2 tablespoons orange zest

1. Combine the wine, orange juice, sugar, cinnamon sticks, and cloves in a large stockpot. Bring to a boil over medium-high heat.

2. Peel the pears, being careful to keep the stems intact. Cut about ½ inch from the bottom of the pears so that they can sit upright in the pot.

3. Holding the stem, gently lower each pear into the boiling wine and set it standing up in the pan. Reduce the heat to low to maintain a bare simmer, and cook for 20 minutes, rotating the pears occasionally to make sure they are turning an even, deep red color.

4. Remove the pan from the heat and cool the pears in the liquid to room temperature. Refrigerate the pears and liquid for at least 4 hours and up to 24 hours.

5. Remove the pears from the liquid. Transfer the liquid to a medium saucepan and boil vigorously over high heat until the sauce is thick and reduced by half.

6. To assemble the dessert, put a dollop of yogurt on a plate, stand the pear in the center of the plate, drizzle with the sauce, and sprinkle with orange zest. Serve immediately.

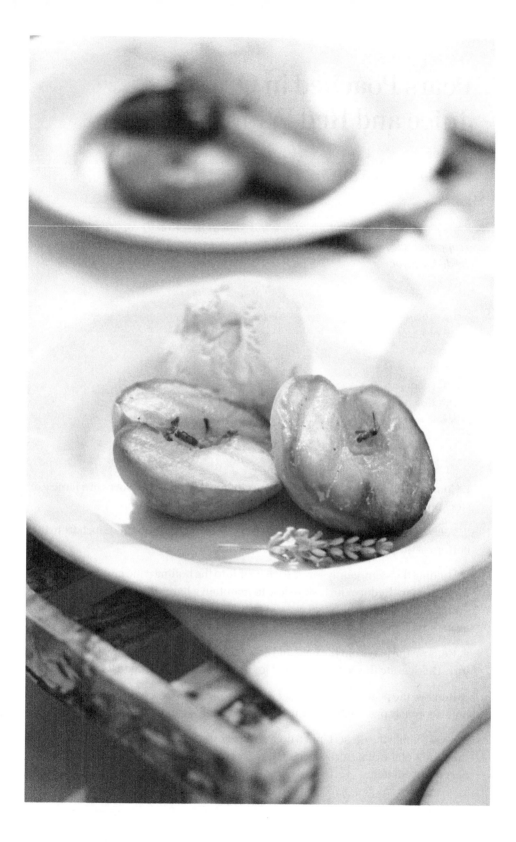

Grilled Peaches

SERVES 4

▸ *CALORIES PER SERVING* **173** // *SODIUM PER SERVING* **5MG**

When peaches meet fire, their natural sugars caramelize into something part peach and part candy. Grilled peaches with no embellishment make a perfect accompaniment to savory dishes like pork or a sweet addition to salads and sandwiches.

1 tablespoon canola oil
1 tablespoon freshly squeezed lemon juice
1 tablespoon honey
4 large peaches, halved
Freshly ground pepper
¼ cup nonfat vanilla yogurt
1 tablespoon lemon zest

1. Preheat an outdoor or stove-top grill to medium-high heat.

2. Whisk together the oil, lemon juice, and honey in a small bowl. With a brush or paper towel, coat the peaches on all sides with the mixture.

3. Grill the peach halves, cut side down, for 3–4 minutes; then turn over and cook the other side for a few minutes. Transfer 2 peach halves to each dessert plate. Season the peaches to taste with pepper.

4. Stir together the yogurt and lemon zest and put a dollop on each plate. Serve immediately.

Clafouti

SERVES 6

▶ *CALORIES PER SERVING* **442** // *SODIUM PER SERVING* **358MG**

Clafouti is a French fruit dessert. Julia Child made it famous, and rightly so. Julia would not like this lightened-up version, though, as her love of milk fat and butter was renowned. She would like, however, that we love clafouti.

Cooking spray
1 pint blueberries, blackberries, pitted Bing cherries, or peach slices
3 large eggs
1 egg yolk
1 cup low-fat milk
1 teaspoon vanilla extract
1 cup sugar
¾ cup whole-wheat flour, sifted
1 teaspoon lemon zest
Pinch of salt
1 tablespoon confectioners' sugar

1. Preheat the oven to 350° F. Thinly coat an 8-inch round cake or springform pan with cooking spray.

2. Spread the fruit in the bottom of the pan.

3. Whisk the eggs, egg yolk, milk, and vanilla together in a large bowl. Continue whisking and gradually add in the sugar, flour, lemon zest, and salt. Continue whisking until the batter is light and airy and the ingredients are well combined.

4. Pour the batter over the fruit and bake for 45 minutes. Cool completely, then invert the pan over a plate and tap out the clafouti. Dust with confectioners' sugar and serve.

Berry Apple Cobbler

SERVES 6

▶ *CALORIES PER SERVING* **267** // *SODIUM PER SERVING* **36MG**

Fruit cobbler is easy and can be made year-round with whatever fruit is in season. This version combines apples and berries, but feel free to add your own favorites, including dried fruits and nuts.

For the cobbler:
1 cup blueberries
1 cup raspberries
2 cups chopped apples
2 tablespoons brown sugar
1 teaspoon ground cinnamon
1 teaspoon lemon zest
1 tablespoon freshly squeezed lemon juice
1½ tablespoons cornstarch

For the topping:
¼ cup whole-wheat flour
¼ cup old-fashioned oats
¼ cup brown sugar
3 tablespoons margarine

1. Preheat the oven to 350° F.

2. In a large bowl, mix all the cobbler ingredients together thoroughly. Transfer to a large baking dish.

3. In a medium bowl, combine the flour, oats, and brown sugar. Work the margarine into the dry ingredients with a fork or pastry cutter until the mixture resembles coarse crumbs. Sprinkle the topping evenly over the fruit.

4. Bake the cobbler for 30–40 minutes, or until brown and bubbly. Serve immediately.

Lighten Up Brownies

SERVES 6, MAKES 1 DOZEN BROWNIES

▶ *CALORIES PER SERVING* **528** // *SODIUM PER SERVING* **178MG**

A world without brownies? Unthinkable! This isn't quite a DASH-friendly recipe because of the use of all-purpose flour, but it is combined with whole-wheat flour to offset its negative effect. The tiny bit of sea salt is important for the chemical reactions needed for the brownie's structure. Crumble bits of brownie over chilled nonfat vanilla yogurt for a "sundae."

Cooking spray
1 large egg
1 large egg white
3 tablespoons nonfat plain yogurt
1½ teaspoons vanilla extract
1½ cups sugar
⅓ cup canola oil
¼ teaspoon sea salt
4 ounces high-quality unsweetened dark baking chocolate, chopped
¼ cup unsweetened cocoa powder
⅓ cup unbleached all-purpose flour
⅓ cup whole-wheat or buckwheat flour

1. Preheat the oven to 375° F. Thinly coat an 8-inch square pan with cooking spray.

2. In a medium bowl, whisk together the egg, egg white, yogurt, and vanilla. Set aside.

3. Combine the sugar, oil, and 3 tablespoons water in a medium saucepan. Stir constantly over medium-high heat for 3 minutes. Remove the pan from the heat. Add the chopped chocolate and cocoa powder. Stir until all the chocolate is melted. Add the all-purpose and whole-wheat flours and stir until smooth. Fold in the egg mixture and stir well to combine.

4. Pour the batter into the pan and bake for 25 minutes. The top should be firm and the interior gooey. Cool the brownies to room temperature, cut into squares, and serve.

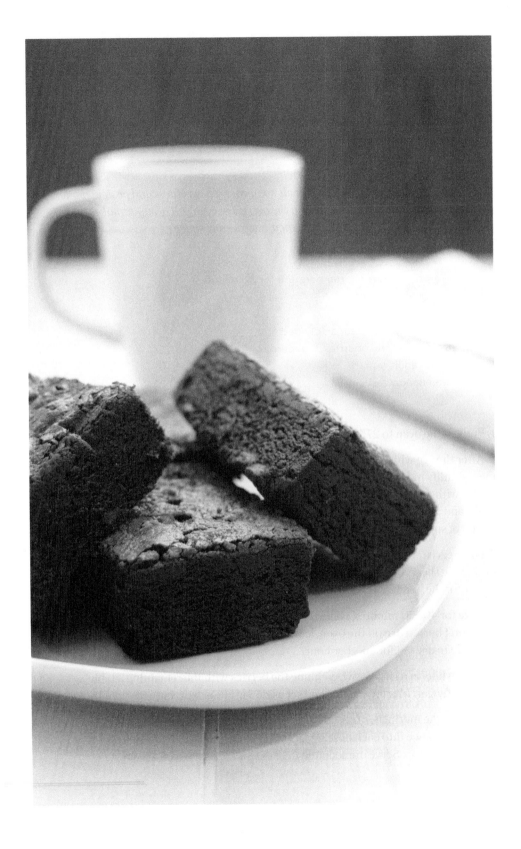

Berries in Meringue

SERVES 6

▸ *CALORIES PER SERVING* **129** // *SODIUM PER SERVING* **107MG**

Meringue is another gift from the French—a miracle of sweetness and protein made with sugar and egg whites. Macerating the berries in a tiny bit of sugar makes them release their natural juices and create their own dessert sauce.

....

3 large egg whites, at room temperature for 30 minutes
½ teaspoon vanilla extract
¼ teaspoon cream of tartar
¾ cup plus 3 tablespoons sugar, divided
3 cups strawberries, raspberries, blueberries, or blackberries
¼ cup nonfat vanilla yogurt
1 tablespoon lemon zest

....

1. Preheat the oven to 275° F. Line a baking sheet with parchment paper.

2. After the egg whites have been at room temperature for 30 minutes (this helps them solidify more quickly) add the vanilla and cream of tartar and beat the egg whites with an electric mixer on high speed. Continue beating until they form soft peaks and appear glossy. While continuing to beat on high speed, gradually add the ¾ cup of sugar in a slow stream until the egg whites form stiff peaks.

3. Form each meringue with 2 heaping tablespoonfuls of egg white dropped on the baking sheet. Use the back of the spoon to smooth it and create a "nest" in the center for the berries. Make 6–8 meringue nests.

4. Bake for 40–50 minutes, checking the meringues frequently near the end so they don't burn. Turn off the oven, leave the door closed, and let the meringues continue to dry out for another hour.

5. Meanwhile, in a large bowl, combine the berries with the remaining 3 tablespoons of sugar. Mix thoroughly and set aside for 1 hour, stirring occasionally.

6. Remove the meringues from the oven and place each on a dessert plate. Spoon berries and sauce into each nest, add a dollop of yogurt on the side, and sprinkle lemon zest on top. Serve immediately.

Homemade Chocolate-Hazelnut Spread

SERVES 4

▸ *CALORIES PER SERVING* **231** // *SODIUM PER SERVING* **17MG; 222MG** *(SEA SALT)*

Chocolate-hazelnut spread is a nutritious treat that turns a piece of fruit or bread into dessert. Fill a platter with fresh and dried fruits to accompany it. If you add the sea salt—which does improve the flavor greatly—note that you will be adding about 200 milligrams of sodium per serving.

1 cup hazelnuts

12 ounces milk chocolate, chopped

2 tablespoons canola or other vegetable oil

3 tablespoons confectioners' sugar

1 tablespoon unsweetened cocoa powder

1 teaspoon vanilla extract

½ teaspoon sea salt (optional)

1. Preheat the oven to 350 degrees F.

2. Spread the hazelnuts in a single layer on a rimmed baking sheet and bake for 10–15 minutes, or until the nuts are toasted and the skins turn dark. Transfer the hazelnuts to a clean kitchen towel and rub roughly with the towel to remove the skins. Set the nuts aside.

3. In the bottom of a double boiler, bring water to a simmer. Put the chocolate in the top part and stir it frequently until melted. Remove the chocolate from the heat.

4. In the bowl of a food processor, combine the hazelnuts, oil, confectioners' sugar, cocoa powder, vanilla, and sea salt, if desired. Process until smooth. Pour in the melted chocolate and pulse until just incorporated into the nut mixture. The spread will keep in an airtight container in the refrigerator for up to 2 weeks.

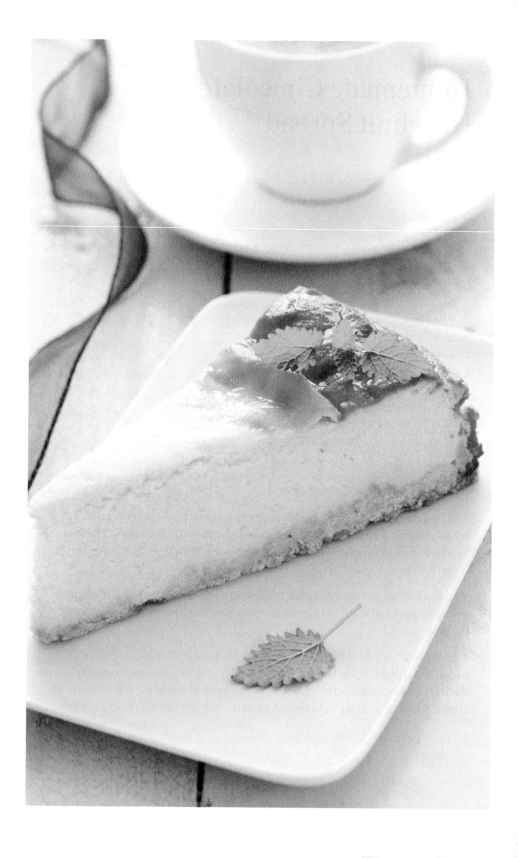

Basic Cheesecake

SERVES 8

▶ *CALORIES PER SERVING* **538** // *SODIUM PER SERVING* **468MG**

Once you have mastered this technique, cheesecake gives the baker a blank canvas upon which to create art. Try topping it with toasted coconut and chopped pecans, melted chocolate and chopped cashew nuts, peanuts and banana chips, or fresh fruit macerated in sugar. The traditional butter has been replaced by coconut or canola oil, with a slight alteration to texture and taste.

1½ cups crushed graham crackers
1 cup plus 3 tablespoons sugar, divided
⅓ coconut or canola oil
1 tablespoon lemon zest
4 (8-ounces) packages low-fat cream cheese, at room temperature
1 teaspoon vanilla extract
4 large eggs

1. Preheat the oven to 325° F.

2. Combine the graham crackers with the 3 tablespoons of sugar, oil, and lemon zest, and stir well. Press the mixture into the bottom of a 9-inch springform pan to form the crust.

3. In a large bowl and using an electric mixer, beat the cream cheese, the remaining 1 cup of sugar, and vanilla together until completely blended. Beating on low speed, add the eggs one at a time, incorporating them completely after each addition. Pour the filling into the crust.

4. Bake for 55 minutes, or until the center of the cheesecake is almost set. Cool slightly, run a knife around the outside of the pan to loosen the cake from the sides, cover, and refrigerate for at least 4 hours before serving.

Chocolate Olive Oil Cake

SERVES 8

▶ *CALORIES PER SERVING* **429** // *SODIUM PER SERVING* **595MG**

For all your extremely healthy eating, you can reward yourself with this extra special treat. Olive oil is a fine fat for baking and it creates a crumb unlike those of most other cakes—it is slightly coarser and beautifully moist.

Cooking spray
3 cups whole-wheat flour
6 tablespoons unsweetened cocoa powder
1 cup sugar
2 teaspoons baking soda
¾ cup extra-virgin olive oil
2 tablespoons apple cider vinegar
1 teaspoon vanilla extract
Pinch of salt
¼ cup confectioners' sugar, for dusting

1. Preheat the oven to 350° F. Thinly coat a 9-inch round cake pan with cooking spray.

2. Whisk together the flour, cocoa powder, sugar, and baking soda. Stir in 2½ cups warm water, the oil, vinegar, vanilla, and salt. Using an electric mixer, beat until the batter is smooth, light, and frothy.

3. Pour the batter into the pan and bake for 30–35 minutes, or until a knife inserted into the center of the cake comes out clean. Cool completely.

4. Remove the cake from the pan, dust with confectioners' sugar, cut into slices, and serve.

Appendix

Shopping and Dining on the DASH Diet

The following guides make eating for good nutrition easier. With these resources in hand, you'll find that following the DASH diet is simple and straightforward, whether eating at home or dining out.

DASH Diet Shopping Tips

When you are on a diet, grocery shopping can be a challenging task. Consider these useful tips to help make your grocery shopping easier and more nutritious.

Shop Around the Edges of the Store

Buy the majority of your foods from the fresh food sections, which are normally located around the edges of the store. This includes fresh fruits and vegetables, fresh meats, seafood, poultry and fresh dairy products.

Skip the Danger Zones

Stay out of the aisles where processed snacks, such as chips and cookies, are located. Out of sight, out of mind.

Read Your Labels

Don't assume that something is low in sodium just because it isn't salty. Read the labels on everything. It's always best to make your food from scratch so that you can control the sodium content, but that isn't possible for everyone. When you need to buy prepared foods, buy those that are lowest in sodium, sugar, and saturated fat. Make note of the best brands so you can eventually shop without having to do any heavy reading.

Buy the Rainbow

To ensure a high intake of antioxidants and micronutrients, choose different kinds of produce every time you shop. Don't just buy green peppers—buy red or orange peppers. Choose lots of dark, leafy greens. Buy fruits that are rich in color, such as watermelon, mango, and dark berries. Consuming a diverse variety of produce will help increase each bite's nutritional value.

Choose Your Meat and Seafood Wisely

Whenever possible, buy organic, grass-fed or pasture-raised meats and wild seafood; they have more omega-3 fats and are more likely to be free of hormones and preservatives. Always choose the leanest cuts of whatever you're buying, and trim visible fat after cooking.

Choose Low-Fat Dairy

Low-fat dairy products should be chosen whenever possible. Cheeses should be nonfat or partially nonfat. Milk should be nonfat or 1 percent fat. Yogurt should be nonfat and low in sugar or sugar-free.

DASH Diet Grocery List

Stock up on the foods you'll need each week. Begin by creating a weekly meal plan with specific recipes; then shop for the ingredients needed to prepare everything on the menu. The following lists contain some of the best foods for creating DASH diet recipes. When shopping for items such as grains, nuts, and dried fruits, seek out a store that offers these items in bulk. You'll find lower prices and often a better selection.

Meats and Seafood

ALLOWED:

- All fish, especially salmon, haddock, mackerel, sardines, and other oily fish
- All shellfish
- Beef: lean steaks and roasts, leanest possible ground meat
- Chicken: skinless and lean ground meat
- Eggs
- Game birds
- Game meats
- Lamb: lean stew meat, steaks, and roasts
- Pork: lean steaks and roasts
- Turkey: skinless and ground breast
- Venison

NOT ALLOWED:

- Bacon, except for low-salt turkey bacon
- Jerky
- Packaged cold cuts and deli meats
- Sausage

Dairy

ALLOWED:

- Almond milk
- Blue cheese
- Cheddar cheese (reduced fat)
- Cottage cheese (low-fat or nonfat)
- Cow's milk (1 percent or nonfat)
- Cream cheese (reduced fat)
- Feta cheese
- Greek yogurt
- Margarine or butter substitute
- Mozzarella cheese
- Parmesan cheese (high in sodium, so limit quantities)
- Provolone cheese (reduced fat)
- Regular yogurt
- Ricotta cheese (reduced fat)
- Sour cream (reduced or nonfat)
- Soy milk
- Swiss cheese

NOT ALLOWED:

- Any full-fat dairy products
- Butter
- Cream

Low-Glycemic Vegetables

ALLOWED:

- Artichoke
- Arugula
- Asparagus
- Avocado
- Bell pepper
- Broccoli
- Brussels sprouts
- Cabbage
- Cauliflower
- Celery
- Collard greens
- Cucumbers
- Eggplant
- Green beans
- Kale
- Lettuce, preferably romaine or dark leafy varieties
- Mushrooms
- Mustard greens
- Onion
- Parsnips
- Radishes
- Snow peas
- Spinach
- Sprouts
- Summer squash
- Swiss chard
- Turnip greens
- Zucchini

High-Glycemic Vegetables

ALLOWED:

- Acorn squash
- Beets
- Butternut squash
- Carrots

- English peas
- Spaghetti squash
- Sweet potato
- Tomato

VERY LIMITED QUANTITIES ALLOWED (ONE SERVING PER WEEK):

- Corn
- White potatoes

Low-Glycemic Fruits

ALLOWED:

- Apple
- Apricot
- Banana
- Blackberries
- Blueberries
- Cantaloupe
- Casaba melon
- Cranberries
- Dates
- Grapes
- Guava
- Honeydew melon
- Lemon
- Lime
- Nectarine
- Papaya
- Peach
- Raspberries
- Rhubarb
- Strawberries
- Watermelon

High-Glycemic Fruits

ALLOWED:

- Cherries
- Figs
- Grapefruit
- Kiwi
- Mango
- Orange
- Pear
- Pineapple

- Plum
- Tangerine
- Watermelon

Fats

ALLOWED:

- Almonds
- Black walnuts
- Brazil nuts
- Canola oil
- Flaxseed oil
- Margarine or butter substitute
- Mayonnaise (low fat)
- Olive oil
- Olives (low sodium)
- Sesame seeds
- Sunflower seeds

NOT ALLOWED:

- All other vegetable oils
- Peanut oil
- Sesame oil

Grains and Dried Legumes

ALLOWED:

- Almond flour
- Amaranth
- Bagels (whole grain)
- Barley
- Beans (black, kidney, pinto, red, and white)
- Black-eyed peas
- Bread (whole grain, preferably very dense)
- Bulgur
- Cereal, cold (whole grain, low carb)
- Cereal, hot (whole grain or mixed grain)
- Chickpeas (garbanzo beans)
- Coconut flour
- Couscous (whole grain)
- English muffins (whole grain)

- Kamut
- Kasha
- Lentils
- Millet
- Quinoa
- Pasta (whole grain)
- Pita (whole grain)
- Rice (brown, red, and wild)
- Spelt
- Split peas
- Steel-cut oats (whole grain)
- Triticale
- Tortillas (whole grain or corn)
- Wheat germ
- Whole-wheat flour

NOT ALLOWED:

- Cornmeal
- Corn muffins or corn bread
- Instant or flavored oatmeal
- Sweetened cold cereals

Condiments, Seasonings, and Miscellaneous

ALLOWED:

- Almond butter
- Applesauce (unsweetened)
- Caesar dressing
- Cashew butter
- Coffee
- Dressings (no or low sodium)
- Flaxseed
- Fruit-only spreads
- Herbs and spices
- Hot sauce
- Iced tea
- Mustard (except honey mustard)
- Peanut butter (in limited quantities)
- Popcorn (air popped)
- Preserves and jellies (no or low sugar)
- Psyllium husk
- Salsa
- Sesame butter (tahini)
- Soup (low sodium)
- Sour or dill pickles
- Soy sauce (low sodium)
- Tea

- Teriyaki sauce (low sodium)
- Tomato or spaghetti sauce (no sugar added, low sodium)
- Vegetable, chicken, or beef broth (no or low sodium)
- Vinegar (apple cider, balsamic, red wine, and rice)
- Vinaigrette
- Whey or soy protein powder (no sugar added)

NOT ALLOWED:

- Mayonnaise (full fat)
- Prepared Alfredo or cheese sauce
- Prepared gravy
- Regular commercial salad dressings
- Regular-sodium steak, barbecue, and other sauces

Sweets

ALLOWED:

- 1-ounce dark chocolate
- Dried fruits (preferably no sugar added)
- Fudge pops (fat-free)
- Frozen fruit bar (no sugar added)
- Gelatin
- Ice cream (low fat)
- Ice pops
- Pudding or pudding cups (fat-free)
- Sorbet or sherbet

Dining Out on the DASH Diet

Dining out is one of life's great pleasures. While it's best to prepare most of the food you eat at home, there are times when you'll want to enjoy a good restaurant. This quick guide will help you make the healthiest choices possible.

Choose Restaurants with Care

If possible, choose restaurants that offer a variety of healthful options. Most restaurants, including an increasing number of fast-food chains, offer at least a few healthful selections, so don't panic if the venue is out of your control. Don't be shy to ask how foods are prepared. Most restaurants are willing to accommodate requests, so ask that they be prepared without added salt, MSG, or salt-containing ingredients.

Remember That Beverages Contain Calories

If you love sugary cocktails such as margaritas or daiquiris, enjoy one and leave it at that. Consider skipping dessert if you've indulged in a calorie-heavy drink. For a festive beverage with half the calories, try filling your glass with half wine and half sparkling water. Remember to sip ice water too. Skip sweet tea, soda, and other sugary drinks to save more calories.

Read Menus Carefully

When reading menus, it helps to know which options are likely to be healthiest. Avoid ordering anything fried, selecting instead offerings that are broiled, baked, blackened, roasted, braised, stewed, poached, or steamed. It is also important to know the terms that indicate high sodium content, for instance: pickled, cured, smoked, soy sauce, and broth. If you are having difficulty selecting a healthful entrée, ask your server for assistance.

Hold the Salt and Ketchup

It is easy to get caught up in the dining experience, and that's okay, but don't let sneaky ingredients throw your diet too off course. Limit condiments, such as mustard, ketchup, pickles, and sauces with salt-containing ingredients. And don't forget the obvious: move the salt shaker away from your plate.

Choose Side Dishes with Care

Rice, mashed potatoes, and fries are all poor choices; so is most restaurant coleslaw. A plain baked potato or sweet potato is a good choice, as are steamed vegetables. If possible choose fruits and vegetables instead of salty snack food.

Eating Dessert?

If you plan to eat dessert, enjoy every bite, but also plan for it as you eat your other courses. The occasional treat is not going to negate all your progress, but be wise in your treat selection. Consider cake without icing, and try to avoid anything with cream filling. The healthiest desserts include baked or poached apples or pears, and fruit pies or cobblers (minus the whipped topping and ice cream). Many restaurants offer low-sugar options as well.

Glossary

Antioxidant: A molecule that inhibits oxidization, alleviating cellular damage and oxidative stress.

Basal metabolic rate (BMR): The number of calories a body at rest requires for basic functioning.

Blood pressure: The pressure that circulating blood exerts upon the walls of arteries and blood vessels.

Body mass index (BMI): A basic measurement of body fat that is used to indicate whether a person is underweight, at a normal weight, overweight, or obese.

Calorie: A single unit of energy-producing potential that is equal to the amount of heat a food is capable of generating. The energy in calories is released when food molecules are digested by the body.

Cardiovascular system: The organ system responsible for blood and lymph circulation throughout the body; includes the heart, arteries, blood vessels, and capillaries.

Cardiovascular disease: A class of diseases that involves the heart, arteries, and/or blood vessels; also known as heart disease.

Carbohydrate: An organic compound that stores energy in various forms, including starches and sugars. Foods that contain high levels of carbohydrates are often referred to as "carbs" or "carbohydrates," even though the foods also contain additional nutrients.

Cholesterol: A lipid fact produced by the liver. Cholesterol is an organic molecule that forms the structures of animal membranes and is essential for every body function.

Cholesterol, HDL: A high-density lipoprotein that aids in the transport of lipids (fats) through the body and which aids in bile creation. HDL cholesterol is also known as "good cholesterol."

Cholesterol, LDL: A low-density lipoprotein that delivers fats to the body's cells, aiding in repairs. When the body's LDL cholesterol level is elevated, the excess cholesterol builds up as plaque inside arteries. For this reason, LDL cholesterol is also known as "bad cholesterol."

Diabetes: A metabolic disease characterized by high blood sugar, caused when the pancreas does not produce a sufficient amount of insulin or when cells fail to respond to the insulin that is produced.

Diet: A structured method of eating, either to maintain weight and health, or to lose weight and improve health.

Emotional eating: Eating to reduce stress or manage other emotions, as opposed to eating when the body signals true hunger.

Fiber, insoluble: Bulky fiber that moves through the digestive system.

Fiber, soluble: Fiber that is absorbed into the bloodstream, where it sweeps lipids away from artery and blood vessel walls.

Glucose: A simple sugar that is absorbed directly into the bloodstream during the digestion process.

Hypertension: Chronic high blood pressure.

Insulin: A type of peptide hormone that is necessary for the regulation of fat and carbohydrate metabolism within the body.

Insulin resistance: A physiological condition characterized by cells that fail to respond appropriately to insulin.

Legume: A plant belonging to the Leguminosae family; the fruits or seeds of these plants, including beans, peas, lentils, and peanuts, are typically referred to as "legumes."

Metabolic syndrome: A combination of medical disorders that, when occurring together, increase an individual's risk of developing diabetes and cardiovascular disease.

Mineral: An earth element that is essential for life.

Obesity: A medical condition characterized by excessive body fat.

Processed food: Food that has been precooked, pulverized, canned, or otherwise prepared and packaged; many processed foods are not considered to be appropriate for consumption by individuals following the DASH diet.

Protein: Large molecules consisting of amino acids that are vital to proper metabolism.

Saturated fat: Fat consisting of triglycerides that contain only saturated fatty acids, and that are typically associated with the development of cardiovascular disease when consumed in excess.

Sedentary lifestyle: A lifestyle that involves restricted movement, whether voluntary or involuntary.

Sodium: A major mineral that is required for healthful fluid balance.

Starch: A carbohydrate containing a high level of glucose.

Stroke: Rapid loss of cerebral function caused by a disturbance in the brain's blood supply.

Sugar: A type of carbohydrate that is rapidly absorbed by the body.

Trans fat: A type of fat that does not occur in nature; it is created during food processing and is associated with coronary heart disease.

Triglyceride: Blood lipids that are typically obtained from vegetable rather than animal sources; though necessary for metabolism, elevated triglyceride levels are associated with heart disease and stroke.

Unsaturated fat: A type of fat that aids in reducing total cholesterol; often referred to as "healthful fat."

Vegan: A person who consumes no animal products.

Vegetarian: A person who consumes no meat, but who may elect to consume fish, shellfish, eggs, and dairy items.

Vitamin: An organic compound that is also a vital nutrient required for bodily function.

Whole grain: A grain that has not been stripped of its bran or germ.

References

Ason, Dan. *DASH Diet SECRETS: Discover New Secrets That Will Change Your Life!* Published by author, 2013. Kindle edition.

Barrett, Patrick. *The Natural Diet: Simple Nutritional Advice for Optimal Health in the Modern World*. Published by author, 2011. Kindle edition.

Benson, Jon, and Andréa Albright. *Thin in 30 Minutes: Walk Your Way Thin in Just 30 Minutes or Less*. McKinney, TX: Fitology/Velocity House, 2012. Kindle edition.

Blatner, Dawn Jackson. *The Flexitarian Diet: The Mostly Vegetarian Way to Lose Weight, Be Healthier, Prevent Disease, and Add Years to Your Life*. New York: McGraw-Hill, 2008.

Esselstyn, Caldwell B., Jr. *Prevent and Reverse Heart Disease: The Revolutionary, Scientifically Proven, Nutrition-Based Cure*. New York: Avery, 2007.

Gillinov, Marc, and Steven Nissen. *Heart 411: The Only Guide to Heart Health You'll Ever Need*. New York: Three Rivers Press, 2012.

Go, Alan S., Dariush Mozaffarian, Véronique L. Roger, Emelia J. Benjamin, Jarret D. Berry, William B. Borden, Dawn M. Bravata, et al. "Heart Disease and Stroke Statistics—2013 Update: A Report from the American Heart Association." On behalf of the American Heart Association Statistics Committee and Stroke Statistics Subcommittee. *Circulation* 127 (2013): e6–e245.

Heller, Marla. *The DASH Diet Action Plan: Proven to Boost Weight Loss and Improve Health*. Northbrook, IL: Amidon Press, 2007.

Heller, Marla. *The DASH Diet Weight Loss Solution: 2 Weeks to Drop Pounds, Boost Metabolism, and Get Healthy*. New York: Grand Central Life and Style, 2012.

Learning Visions. *The DASH Diet Solution and 60 Day Weight Loss and Fitness Journal*. Thousand Oaks, CA: Learning Vision, 2013.

Moore, Thomas J., Megan C. Murphy, and Mark Jenkins. *The DASH Diet for Weight Loss: Lose Weight and Keep It Off—the Healthy Way—with America's Most Respected Diet*. New York: Gallery Books, 2012.

Moore, Thomas J., Laura Svetkey, Pao-Hwa Lin, Njeri Karanja, and Mark Jenkins. *The DASH Diet for Hypertension: Lower Your Blood Pressure in 14 Days—without Drugs*. New York: Pocket Books, 2003.

Nestle, Marion. *What to Eat*. New York: North Point Press, 2006.

Robinson, Stephen. *How to Use the DASH Diet to Lose Weight for Good*. UK Kindle Creations, 2013. Kindle edition.

Spencer, Stan. *The Diet Dropout's Guide to Natural Weight Loss: Find Your Easiest Path to Naturally Thin*. Riverside, CA: Fine Life Books, 2013. Kindle edition.

Index

A

Acorn Squash, Apple, and
Peach "Pie," 103
Additives in DASH diet, 46–47
Alcoholic beverages, 6
Alfalfa sprouts
Cilantro-Avocado Tea
Sandwiches, 213
Tiny Turkey Quesadillas,
218–219
Almond milk
Chocolate Pudding, 290–291
Green Tea and Banana
Smoothie, 90
Almonds
Cherries, Almonds,
and Cheese, 281
Dark Chocolate Almond
Clusters, 294–295
Sweet-Hot Maple
Almonds, 190
Almost Mexican Pita, 150–151
Appetite, 6
Appetizers. See Snacks and
appetizers
Apples
Acorn Squash, Apple, and
Peach "Pie," 103
Baked Applesauce with
Walnuts, 199
Berry Apple Cobbler, 307
Boneless Pork Chops with
Curried Apples, 266
Crunchy Chicken Salad, 140
Green Monster, The, 92–93
Apricots
Bobotie Lite, 178
Agua Fresca, 184–185
Argentinean-Style Flank Steak, 268

Arugula
Creamy Beans and Greens, 232
Flattened Chicken on Arugula
Salad, 139
Avocado
Chocolate Pudding, 290–291
Cilantro-Avocado Tea
Sandwiches, 213
Cold Avocado and Shrimp
Soup, 145
DASH Migas, 116
Green Monster, The, 92–93
Soft Beef Tacos, 176–177
Substantial Fruit Salad, 98
Tiny Turkey Quesadillas,
218–219

B

Baked Applesauce with Walnuts,
199
Baked Chili-Lime Tortilla Chips,
198
Baked Eggs with Truffle Oil and
Fontina Cheese, 109
Baking, 61
Balsamic Berries, 288
Bananas
Chocolate Pudding, 290–291
Green Tea and Banana
Smoothie, 90
Mango Blast Smoothie, 88–89
Red, White, and Blue Fruit
Kebabs, 186
Stomach Soother
Smoothie, The, 91
Yogurt and Tropical Fruit
Parfaits, 96–97
Barbecuing, 61
Basal metabolic rate, defined, 26–27

Basic Cheesecake, 313
Basil
Pasta with Basil or Cilantro
Pesto, 236–237
Strawberry and Cream Cheese
Cakes, 121
Strawberry-Mango Salsa with
Basil, 200–201
Beans. See specific
Beef. See also Ground beef
Argentinean-Style Flank
Steak, 268
Filet Mignon with Red Wine
au Jus, 179–181
Pot Roast with Sweet Potatoes,
Peas, and Onions, 269–271
Soft Beef Tacos, 176–177
Vegetable Beef Stew, 230–231
Beets
Vegetable Chips, 196–197
Bell pepper
Breakfast Hash, 127
Bulgar with Vegetables and
Goat Cheese, 233
Coconut Fish Stew, 228
Cold Soba Noodles with Peanut
Sauce, 160–161
DASH Migas, 116
Easy Breakfast Casserole with
Vegetables, 113
Egg Tart with Sweet Potato
Crust, 118–120
Folded French Omelet,
104–105
Mini Crab Cakes on Baby
Greens, 162–163
Niçoise-Style Salad, 132–134
Quick Vegetarian Ramen
Noodle Soup, 226–227

Roasted Red Pepper Dip,
206–207
Roasted Vegetables on Ciabatta,
154–155
Shrimp and Mango
"Ceviche," 216
Spanish-Style Scrambled
Eggs, 108
Spicy Tofu Stir-Fry, 244
Turkey and Rice–Stuffed
Peppers, 252
Vegetable and Mozzarella
Frittata, 146–148
Berries. See specific
Berries in Meringue, 310
Berry Apple Cobbler, 307
Best Practices Roast Chicken,
256–257
Beta glucan, 102
Beverages. See also Smoothies
Agua Fresca, 184
Soy Milk Shakes, 280
Black beans
Turkey Chili with Black
Beans, 229
Blackberries
Berries in Meringue, 310
Clafouti, 306
Vanilla and Lemon Berry
Parfaits, 286–287
Blueberries
Balsamic Berries, 288
Berries in Meringue, 310
Berry Apple Cobbler, 307
Clafouti, 306
Fruit Sauce for Sundaes, 284
Peach Berry Fizz, 94
Red, White, and Blue Fruit
Kebabs, 186
Sweet Potato Oatmeal, 100–101
Vanilla and Lemon Berry
Parfaits, 286–287
Bobotie Lite, 178
Bocconcini
Pasta Caprese, 158–159
Turkey Mozzarella
Shooters, 217
Body mass index (BMI)
defined, 25
determining your, 36–37
Boneless Pork Chops with Curried
Apples, 266
Bread. See Ciabatta bread;
Multigrain bread;
Whole-wheat bread
Breakfast Burrito, 124–125
Breakfast Hash, 127

Breakfasts, 87–129
Acorn Squash, Apple, and Peach
"Pie," 103
Baked Eggs with Truffle Oil and
Fontina Cheese, 109
Breakfast Burrito, 124–125
Breakfast Hash, 127
Creamy "French" Scrambled
Eggs, 107
Crustless Spinach Quiche,
114–115
Cucumber and Ricotta Open-
Face Sandwiches, 122
DASH Migas, 116
Easy Breakfast Casserole with
Vegetables, 113
Egg Tart with Sweet Potato
Crust, 118–120
Egg White Omelet, 106
Folded French Omelet,
104–105
Fruit-Filled French Toast, 126
Granola, Your Way, 102
Green Monster, The, 92–93
Green Tea and Banana
Smoothie, 90
Grits and Eggs, 117
Hollywood Broiled
Grapefruit, 95
Homemade Breakfast Sausage,
Three Ways, 128–129
Hummus and Sardines on
Toast, 123
Mango Blast Smoothie, 88–89
Oatmeal with Pistachios and
Currants, 99
Peach Berry Fizz, 94
Perfect Poached Eggs with
Lemon Sauce, 110–112
Spanish-Style Scrambled
Eggs, 108
Stomach Soother
Smoothie, The, 91
Strawberry and Cream
Cheese Cakes, 121
Substantial Fruit Salad, 98
Sweet Potato Oatmeal, 100–101
Yogurt and Tropical Fruit
Parfaits, 96–97
Broccoli
Bulgar with Vegetables and
Goat Cheese, 233
Cold Soba Noodles with Peanut
Sauce, 160–161
Easy Breakfast Casserole with
Vegetables, 113
Lightning-Fast Chicken
Stir-Fry, 171

Broiling, 60
Brown rice
Chicken Breasts with Citrus
and Chili Sauce on Coconut
Rice, 258–259
Chicken Breasts with Mango-
Rosemary Sauce on
Brown Rice, 262
Chicken Curry, 172–174
Lightning-Fast Chicken
Stir-Fry, 171
Turkey and Rice–Stuffed
Peppers, 252
Bulgar with Vegetables and
Goat Cheese, 233
Burrito, Breakfast, 124–125

C

Caffeine, 6, 11
Cajun Popcorn, 191
Calories
daily requirements, 27–28
tips for reducing intake, 39
Candied Pecans, 293
Cannellini beans
White Bean and Sage Soup, 141
Cantaloupe
Cantaloupe Granita, 276
Melon Soup with Mint and
Yogurt, 144
Cardiovascular benefits, 30–31
Carrots
Massaged Kale Salad, 138
Quick Vegetarian Ramen
Noodle Soup, 226–227
Turkey Bolognese, 242–243
Vegetable and Hummus
Pita, 152
Vegetable Beef Stew, 230–231
Celery
Vegetable Smoothie, 192–193
Challah
Creamy "French" Scrambled
Eggs, 107
Fruit-Filled French Toast, 126
Cheddar cheese
Breakfast Burrito, 124–125
Easy Breakfast Casserole with
Vegetables, 113
Egg Tart with Sweet Potato
Crust, 118–120
Cherries
Cherries, Almonds, and Cheese,
281
Clafouti, 306
Hollywood Broiled
Grapefruit, 95

Cherry tomatoes
  Bulgar with Vegetables and
    Goat Cheese, 233
  Layered Vegetable
    Casserole, 234
  Lemon-Scented Chicken
    Kebabs on Saffron Rice,
    253–254
  Quinoa with Vegetables and
    Toasted Pecans, 156–157
  Vegetable Smoothie, 192–193
Chia seeds
  Oatmeal with Pistachios and
    Currants, 99
  Peach Berry Fizz, 94
  Sweet Potato Oatmeal, 100–101
Chicken
  Almost Mexican Pita, 150–151
  Best Practices Roast Chicken,
    256–257
  Chicken Breasts with Citrus
    and Chili Sauce on Coconut
    Rice, 258–259
  Chicken Breasts with Mango-
    Rosemary Sauce on
    Brown Rice, 262
  Chicken Breast with Mushroom
    Sauce on Wild Rice,
    260–261
  Chicken Curry, 172–174
  Crunchy Chicken Salad, 140
  Flattened Chicken on Arugula
    Salad, 139
  Homemade Breakfast Sausage,
    Three Ways, 128–129
  Lemon-Glazed Tiny
    Drumsticks, 220
  Lemon-Scented Chicken
    Kebabs on Saffron Rice,
    253–254
  Lightning-Fast Chicken
    Stir-Fry, 171
  Panko-Crusted Chicken Strips
    with Apricot Dipping
    Sauce, 255
Chickpeas
  Homemade Hummus with
    Crudités, 209
  Spicy Chickpeas and
    Turkey, 167–168
  Spicy Oil-Roasted
    Chickpeas, 208
Chile pepper
  Chicken Breasts with Citrus
    and Chili Sauce on Coconut
    Rice, 258–259
  Spicy Tofu Stir-Fry, 244
Chili, Turkey, with Black Beans, 229

Chocolate
  Chocolate Olive Oil Cake, 314
  Chocolate Pudding, 290–291
  Dark Chocolate Almond
    Clusters, 294–295
  Dark Chocolate–Covered
    Fruits, 302
  Frozen Chocolate Cannoli
    Sandwiches, 292
  Heart-Healing Chocolate Chip
    Cookies, 298–300
  Homemade Chocolate-
    Hazelnut Spread, 311
  Lighten Up Brownies, 308–309
  Meringue Kisses, 301
Ciabatta bread
  Bobotie Lite, 178
  Cucumber and Ricotta Open-
    Face Sandwiches, 122
  Hummus and Sardines on
    Toast, 123
  Roasted Vegetables on Ciabatta,
    154–155
Cilantro
  Cilantro-Avocado Tea
    Sandwiches, 213
  Pasta with Basil or Cilantro
    Pesto, 236–237
Clafouti, 306
Coconut Fish Stew, 228
Coconut milk
  Coconut Fish Stew, 228
  Cold Soba Noodles with Peanut
    Sauce, 160–161
Coconut Soup, 289
Coconut water
  Chicken Breasts with Citrus
    and Chili Sauce on Coconut
    Rice, 258–259
Cold Avocado and Shrimp Soup,
  145
Cold Soba Noodles with Peanut
  Sauce, 160–161
Collard greens
  Vegetable Chips, 196–197
Cooking methods, DASH-friendly,
  59–61
Cookware, selecting the right, 59
Corn
  Layered Vegetable
    Casserole, 234
  Louisiana Shrimp Boil,
    249–251
  Soft Beef Tacos, 176–177
Corned beef
  Breakfast Hash, 127
Cottage cheese
  Easy Breakfast Casserole with
    Vegetables, 113

Crabmeat
  Mini Crab Cakes on Baby
    Greens, 162–163
  Onion and Herb Dip, 204–205
Cranberries
  Agua Fresca, 164–165
  Massaged Kale Salad, 138
  Sweet Potato Oatmeal, 100–101
Cream cheese
  Basic Cheesecake, 313
  Cucumber and Dill Tea
    Sandwiches, 215
  Perfect Poached Eggs with
    Lemon Sauce, 110–112
  Strawberry and Cream Cheese
    Cakes, 121
Creamy Beans and Greens, 232
Creamy "French" Scrambled
  Eggs, 107
Crunchy Chicken Salad, 140
Crustless Spinach Quiche, 114–115
Cucumbers. See also English
  cucumbers
  Cold Avocado and Shrimp
    Soup, 145
  Cucumber and Dill Tea
    Sandwiches, 215
  Cucumber and Ricotta Open-
    Face Sandwiches, 122
  Cucumber Gazpacho, 194
  Niçoise-Style Salad, 132–134
  Noodle Salad with Shrimp and
    Cucumber, 166
  Vegetable and Hummus
    Pita, 152
  Vietnamese Pork
    Sandwiches, 175
Currants
  Oatmeal with Pistachios and
    Currants, 99
  Quinoa with Vegetables and
    Toasted Pecans, 156–157

D

Dairy products
  choosing low-fat, 316
  low-fat, in DASH diet, 44–45
Dark Chocolate Almond Clusters,
  294–295
Dark Chocolate–Covered
  Fruits, 302
DASH diet
  basic guidelines, 5
  dining out on the, 322–324
  eating guide for, 55–58
  effect on health, 13–16
  exercise and, 28–29

fats, oils, and other additives
in, 46–47
fruits in, 44
grains in, 43
grocery list for, 316–322
low-fat dairy products in,
44–45
meat, poultry, fish, eggs, and
vegetable proteins in,
45–46
nuts, seeds, and legumes in, 45
off-limit foods in, 5–6
for optimal health, 30–32
origin of, 3
pairing with other diets, 8
prevention and reversal of
prediabetes and heart
disease, 14–15
reasons for choosing, 7–8
science behind, 12–13
servings in, 4
shopping tips for, 315–316
tips for planning your, 35–42
vegetables in, 44
for weight loss, 24–29
DASH-friendly cooking methods,
59–61
DASH Meatballs, 222–223
DASH Migas, 116
Desserts, 273–324
Balsamic Berries, 288
Basic Cheesecake, 313
Berries in Meringue, 310
Berry Apple Cobbler, 307
Candied Pecans, 293
Cantaloupe Granita, 276
Cherries, Almonds, and
Cheese, 281
Chocolate Olive Oil Cake, 314
Chocolate Pudding, 290–291
Clafouti, 306
Coconut Soup, 289
Dark Chocolate Almond
Clusters, 294–295
Dark Chocolate–Covered
Fruits, 302
Fig Cookies, 297
Figs Baked with Goat Cheese
and Honey, 296
Frozen Chocolate Cannoli
Sandwiches, 292
Fruit Sauce for Sundaes, 284
Grilled Peaches, 304–305
Heart-Healing Chocolate Chip
Cookies, 298–300
Herbed Grapefruit Sorbet, 277
Homemade Chocolate-
Hazelnut Spread, 311

Lemonade Ice Pops, 278–279
Lighten Up Brownies, 308–309
Meringue Kisses, 301
Pears Poached in Orange Juice
and Red Wine, 303
Rhubarb Compote, 285
Soy Milk Shakes, 280
Tea and Jam Platter, 282–283
Vanilla and Lemon Berry
Parfaits, 286–287
Watermelon Ice, 274–275
Dietary Approaches to Stop
Hypertension (DASH).
See DASH diet
Dietary intake guidelines,
conformity with accepted,
31–32
Dill
Cucumber and Dill Tea
Sandwiches, 215
Dining out
on the DASH diet, 322–324
planning ahead for, 50
Dinners, 225–271
Argentinean-Style Flank
Steak, 268
Best Practices Roast Chicken,
256–257
Boneless Pork Chops with
Curried Apples, 266
Bulgar with Vegetables and
Goat Cheese, 233
Chicken Breasts with Citrus
and Chili Sauce on Coconut
Rice, 258–259
Chicken Breasts with Mango-
Rosemary Sauce on Brown
Rice, 262
Chicken Breasts with
Mushroom Sauce on
Wild Rice, 260–261
Coconut Fish Stew, 228
Creamy Beans and Greens, 232
Grilled Pork Tenderloin with
Garlic and Herbs, 264–265
Kale and Tomatoes on Whole-
Wheat Pasta, 235
Layered Vegetable
Casserole, 234
Lemon-Scented Chicken
Kebabs on Saffron Rice,
253–254
Louisiana Shrimp Boil,
249–251
Panko-Crusted Chicken
Strips with Apricot
Dipping Sauce, 255

Pan-Seared Whitefish on
Lemony Quinoa, 245
Pasta with Basil or Cilantro
Pesto, 236–237
Perfect Pan-Seared Fish,
246–247
Portobello Stroganoff over Egg
Noodles, 238
Pot Roast with Sweet Potatoes,
Peas, and Onions, 269–271
Quick Vegetarian Ramen
Noodle Soup, 226–227
Scottish Meatloaf, 267
Shrimp with Jalapeño-Orange
Sauce over Pasta, 248
Spicy Tofu Stir-Fry, 244
Turkey and Rice–Stuffed
Peppers, 252
Turkey Bolognese, 242–243
Turkey Chili with Black
Beans, 229
Vegetable Beef Stew, 230–231
Vegetable Lasagna, 239–241
Winemaker's Feast, The, 263
Dips
Onion and Herb Dip, 204–205
Roasted Red Pepper Dip,
206–207

E

Easy Breakfast Casserole with
Vegetables, 113
Eating, intentional, 57–58
Eating guide for DASH diet, 55–58
Eating habits, creating healthful,
55–57
Eating issues, addressing
emotional, 49
Edamame, 188
Spiced Edamame, 188–189
Egg noodles
Boneless Pork Chops with
Curried Apples, 266
Portobello Stroganoff over Egg
Noodles, 238
Winemaker's Feast, The, 263
Eggplant
Layered Vegetable
Casserole, 234
Roasted Vegetables on Ciabatta,
154–155
Vegetable Lasagna, 239–241
Vegetable Napoleons, 149
Eggs
Baked Eggs with Truffle Oil and
Fontina Cheese, 109

Basic Cheesecake, 313
Bobotie Lite, 178
Breakfast Burrito, 124–125
Clafouti, 306
Creamy "French" Scrambled
    Eggs, 107
Crustless Spinach Quiche,
    114–115
in DASH diet, 45–46
DASH Migas, 116
Easy Breakfast Casserole with
    Vegetables, 113
Egg Tart with Sweet Potato
    Crust, 118–120
Folded French Omelet,
    104–105
Fruit-Filled French Toast, 126
Herbed Deviled Eggs, 210–211
Niçoise-Style Salad, 132–134
Perfect Poached Eggs with
    Lemon Sauce, 110–112
Spanish-Style Scrambled
    Eggs, 108
Egg whites
Berries in Meringue, 310
Egg White Omelet, 106
Fig Cookies, 297
Homemade Breakfast Sausage,
    Three Ways, 128–129
Lighten Up Brownies, 308–309
Meringue Kisses, 301
English cucumbers
Cucumber Gazpacho, 194
Pickled Cucumbers, 195
English muffins
Baked Eggs with Truffle Oil and
    Fontina Cheese, 109
Turkey Burgers with
    Cranberry-Scallion Sauce,
    169–170
Exercise
DASH diet and, 28–29
making time to, 49

F
Fats in DASH diet, 46–47
Feta cheese
Vegetable Napoleons, 149
Watermelon, Feta, and Mint
    Summer Salad, 136–167
Figs
Fig Cookies, 297
Figs Baked with Goat Cheese
    and Honey, 296
Filet Mignon with Red Wine au Jus,
    179–181

Fish and seafood. See also Lobster;
    Salmon; Shrimp
choosing wisely, 316
Coconut Fish Stew, 228
in DASH diet, 45–46
Pan-Seared Whitefish on
    Lemony Quinoa, 245
Perfect Pan-Seared Fish,
    246–247
Flattened Chicken on Arugula
    Salad, 139
Flaxseed
Oatmeal with Pistachios and
    Currants, 99
Peach Berry Fizz, 94
Folded French Omelet, 104–105
Fontina Cheese, Baked Eggs with
    Truffle Oil and, 109
Food and exercise diary, keeping, 49
Food pushers, saying no to, 50
Foods
eliminating undesirable, 39–41
emphasis on whole, healthful,
    21–22
high-sodium, 16
off-limits, 5–6
French Toast, Fruit-Filled, 126
Frittata, Vegetable and Mozzarella,
    146–148
Frozen Chocolate Cannoli
    Sandwiches, 292
Fruit-Filled French Toast, 126
Fruits. See also specific fruits
in DASH diet, 44
Fruit Sauce for Sundaes, 284
Fullness, 6

G
Gazpacho, Cucumber, 194
Ginger
Stomach Soother
    Smoothie, The, 91
Goals, setting attainable, 38
Goat cheese
Bulgar with Vegetables and
    Goat Cheese, 233
Figs Baked with Goat Cheese
    and Honey, 296
Graham crackers
Basic Cheesecake, 313
Frozen Chocolate Cannoli
    Sandwiches, 292
Grains in DASH diet, 43
Granola, Your Way, 102
Grapefruit
Dark Chocolate–Covered
    Fruits, 302

Herbed Grapefruit Sorbet, 277
Hollywood Broiled
    Grapefruit, 95
Grapes
Crunchy Chicken Salad, 140
Winemaker's Feast, The, 263
Grape tomatoes
Cucumber Gazpacho, 194
Kale and Tomatoes on
    Whole-Wheat Pasta, 235
Green beans
Niçoise-Style Salad, 132–134
Green Monster, The, 92–93
Greens
Vegetable and Mozzarella
    Frittata, 146–148
Green Tea and Banana
    Smoothie, 90
Grilled Peaches, 304–305
Grilled Pork Tenderloin with Garlic
    and Herbs, 264–265
Grilling, 61
Grits and Eggs, 117
Grocery list for DASH diet,
    316–322
Ground beef
Bobotie Lite, 178
DASH Meatballs, 222–223
Scottish Meatloaf, 267
Gruyère
Crustless Spinach Quiche,
    114–115

H
Health
effect of DASH diet on, 13–16
keeping choices available, 50
30-day meal plan for, 62–84
Heart disease, DASH diet and,
    14–15
Heart-Healing Chocolate Chip
    Cookies, 298–300
Herbed Deviled Eggs, 210–211
Herbed Grapefruit Sorbet, 277
Herbs
Egg White Omelet, 106
Vegetable and Mozzarella
    Frittata, 146–148
High blood pressure, reducing
    sodium in alleviating, 19
Hollywood Broiled Grapefruit, 95
Homemade Breakfast Sausage,
    Three Ways, 128–129
Homemade Chocolate-Hazelnut
    Spread, 311
Homemade Hummus with
    Crudités, 209

Homemade Tomato Soup, 142–143
Honey
    Acorn Squash, Apple, and
      Peach "Pie," 103
    Fruit-Filled French Toast, 126
    Granola, Your Way, 102
    Green Tea and Banana
      Smoothie, 90
    Hollywood Broiled
      Grapefruit, 95
    Melon Soup with Mint and
      Yogurt, 144
    Oatmeal with Pistachios and
      Currants, 99
    Stomach Soother
      Smoothie, The, 91
    Strawberry and Cream Cheese
      Cakes, 121
    Substantial Fruit Salad, 98
    Sweet Potato Oatmeal,
      100–101
Honeydew melon
    Green Tea and Banana
      Smoothie, 90
Hummus
    Homemade Hummus with
      Crudités, 209
    Hummus and Sardines on
      Toast, 123
    Vegetable and Hummus
      Pita, 152
Hypertension, understanding,
    19–21

I

Intentional eating, 57–58

J

Jalapeño peppers
    Louisiana Shrimp Boil,
      249–251
    Roasted Red Pepper Dip,
      206–207
    Shrimp and Mango
      "Ceviche," 216
    Shrimp with Jalapeño-Orange
      Sauce over Pasta, 248
    Strawberry-Mango Salsa with
      Basil, 200–201
    Thai Pork in Lettuce
      Wraps, 221
    Tomato Salsa with Jalapeños
      and Lime, 203
    Vegetable Smoothie, 192–193

K

Kale
    Green Monster, The, 92–93
    Kale and Tomatoes on Whole-
      Wheat Pasta, 235
    Massaged Kale Salad, 138
Kebabs
    Lemon-Scented Chicken
      Kebabs on Saffron Rice,
      253–254
    Red, White, and Blue Fruit
      Kebabs, 186
Kidney beans
    Creamy Beans and Greens, 232

L

Labels, reading, 315–316
Lasagna noodles
    Vegetable Lasagna, 239–241
Layered Vegetable Casserole, 234
Legumes in DASH diet, 45
Lemonade Ice Pops, 278–279
Lemon curd
    Vanilla and Lemon Berry
      Parfaits, 286–287
Lemon-Glazed Tiny
    Drumsticks, 220
Lemons
    Lemonade Ice Pops, 278–279
    Lemon-Scented Chicken
      Kebabs on Saffron Rice,
      253–254
    Simple Rosemary Salmon,
      164–165
Lettuce. *See also* Romaine lettuce
    Crunchy Chicken Salad, 140
    Niçoise-Style Salad, 132–134
    Orange, Avocado, and Shrimp
      Salad, 135
    Shrimp and Mango
      "Ceviche," 216
    Thai Pork in Lettuce Wraps, 221
    Vegetable and Hummus
      Pita, 152
    Wild Salmon Salad Pita, 153
Lighten Up Brownies, 308–309
Lightning-Fast Chicken Stir-Fry, 171
Limes, Tomato Salsa with
    Jalapeños and, 203
Lobster
    Simple Lobster Tea
      Sandwiches, 214
Louisiana Shrimp Boil, 249–251
Lunches, 131–181
    Almost Mexican Pita, 150–151
    Bobotie Lite, 178

Chicken Curry, 172–174
Cold Avocado and Shrimp
    Soup, 145
Cold Soba Noodles with Peanut
    Sauce, 160–161
Crunchy Chicken Salad, 140
Filet Mignon with Red Wine au
    Jus, 179–181
Flattened Chicken on Arugula
    Salad, 139
Homemade Tomato Soup,
    142–143
Lightning-Fast Chicken
    Stir-Fry, 171
Massaged Kale Salad, 138
Melon Soup with Mint and
    Yogurt, 144
Mini Crab Cakes on Baby
    Greens, 162–163
Niçoise-Style Salad, 132–134
Noodle Salad with Shrimp and
    Cucumber, 166
Orange, Avocado, and Shrimp
    Salad, 135
Pasta Caprese, 158–159
Quinoa with Vegetables and
    Toasted Pecans, 156–157
Roasted Vegetables on Ciabatta,
    154–155
Simple Rosemary Salmon,
    164–165
Soft Beef Tacos, 176–177
Spicy Chickpeas and Turkey,
    167–168
Turkey Burgers with
    Cranberry-Scallion Sauce,
    169–170
Vegetable and Hummus
    Pita, 152
Vegetable and Mozzarella
    Frittata, 146–148
Vegetable Napoleons, 149
Vietnamese Pork
    Sandwiches, 175
Watermelon, Feta, and Mint
    Summer Salad, 136–137
White Bean and Sage Soup, 141
Wild Salmon Salad Pita, 153

M

Mango
    Chicken Breasts with
      Mango-Rosemary Sauce
      on Brown Rice, 262
    Mango Blast Smoothie, 88–89
    Shrimp and Mango
      "Ceviche," 216

Strawberry-Mango Salsa with
Basil, 200–201
Yogurt and Tropical Fruit
Parfaits, 96–97
Maple syrup
Chocolate Pudding, 290–291
Sweet-Hot Maple Almonds, 190
Massaged Kale Salad, 138
Meatballs, DASH, 222–223
Meatloaf, Scottish, 267
Meats
choosing wisely, 316
in DASH diet, 45–46
Melon Soup with Mint and
Yogurt, 144
Meringue Kisses, 301
Metabolic syndrome, relief from,
7–8
Mind-body connection, 57–58
Mini Crab Cakes on Baby Greens,
162–163
Mint
Melon Soup with Mint and
Yogurt, 144
Watermelon, Feta, and Mint
Summer Salad, 136–167
Mistakes, forgiving, 51
Monterey jack cheese
Almost Mexican Pita, 150–151
Mozzarella cheese
Layered Vegetable
Casserole, 234
Turkey Mozzarella Shooters, 217
Vegetable and Mozzarella
Frittata, 146–148
Vegetable Lasagna, 239–241
Multigrain bread
Creamy "French" Scrambled
Eggs, 107
Fruit-Filled French Toast, 126
Mushrooms
Chicken Breast with Mushroom
Sauce on Wild Rice,
260–261
Portobello Stroganoff over Egg
Noodles, 238
Quick Vegetarian Ramen
Noodle Soup, 226–227
Vegetable and Mozzarella
Frittata, 146–148

N

Navel oranges
Orange, Avocado, and Shrimp
Salad, 135
Niçoise-Style Salad, 132–134

Noodle Salad with Shrimp and
Cucumber, 166
Nutrition, daily breakdown, 5
Nuts. See also specific
in DASH diet, 45
Granola, Your Way, 102

O

Oat flour
Heart-Healing Chocolate Chip
Cookies, 298–300
Oatmeal with Pistachios and
Currants, 99
Oats
Berry Apple Cobbler, 307
Granola, Your Way, 102
Heart-Healing Chocolate Chip
Cookies, 298–300
Oatmeal with Pistachios and
Currants, 99
Scottish Meatloaf, 267
Sweet Potato Oatmeal, 100–101
Oils in DASH diet, 46–47
Omelets
Egg White Omelet, 106
Folded French Omelet,
104–105
Onions
Bobotie Lite, 178
Breakfast Hash, 127
Crustless Spinach Quiche,
114–115
Egg Tart with Sweet Potato
Crust, 118–120
Onion and Herb Dip, 204–205
Portobello Stroganoff over Egg
Noodles, 238
Scottish Meatloaf, 267
Spanish-Style Scrambled
Eggs, 108
Substantial Fruit Salad, 98
Turkey Bolognese, 242–243
Turkey Chili with Black
Beans, 229
Vegetable Beef Stew, 230–231
White Bean and Sage Soup, 141
Oranges
Dark Chocolate–Covered
Fruits, 302
Lemonade Ice Pops, 278–279
Orange, Avocado, and Shrimp
Salad, 135
Red, White, and Blue Fruit
Kebabs, 186
Simple Rosemary Salmon,
164–165
Yogurt and Tropical Fruit
Parfaits, 96–97

P

Panko-Crusted Chicken Strips with
Apricot Dipping Sauce, 255
Pan-Seared Whitefish on Lemony
Quinoa, 245
Papaya
Yogurt and Tropical Fruit
Parfaits, 96–97
Pasta, whole-wheat
Kale and Tomatoes on Whole-
Wheat Pasta, 235
Noodle Salad with Shrimp and
Cucumber, 166
Pasta Caprese, 158–159
Pasta with Basil or Cilantro
Pesto, 236–237
Shrimp with Jalapeño-Orange
Sauce over Pasta, 248
Turkey Bolognese, 242–243
Pasta Caprese, 158–159
Pasta with Basil or Cilantro Pesto,
236–237
Peach Berry Fizz, 94
Peaches
Acorn Squash, Apple, and
Peach "Pie," 103
Clafouti, 306
Grilled Peaches, 304–305
Peach Berry Fizz, 94
Substantial Fruit Salad, 98
Peanut butter
Cold Soba Noodles with Peanut
Sauce, 160–161
Pears Poached in Orange Juice and
Red Wine, 303
Peas
Pot Roast with Sweet Potatoes,
Peas, and Onions, 269–271
Vegetable Beef Stew, 230–231
Pecans
Candied Pecans, 293
Quinoa with Vegetables and
Toasted Pecans, 156–157
Perfect Pan-Seared Fish, 246–247
Perfect Poached Eggs with Lemon
Sauce, 110–112
Physical, treating yourself to a, 38
Pickled Cucumbers, 195
Pineapple
Dark Chocolate–Covered
Fruits, 302
Substantial Fruit Salad, 98
Watermelon Ice, 274–275
Pistachios
Oatmeal with Pistachios and
Currants, 99
Watermelon and Pistachio
Salad, 202

Pitas
    Almost Mexican Pita, 150–151
    Vegetable and Hummus
        Pita, 152
    Wild Salmon Salad Pita, 153
Poaching, 60
Popcorn, Cajun, 191
Pork
    Boneless Pork Chops with
        Curried Apples, 266
    Grilled Pork Tenderloin with
        Garlic and Herbs, 264–265
    Homemade Breakfast Sausage,
        Three Ways, 128–129
    Thai Pork in Lettuce Wraps, 221
    Vietnamese Pork
        Sandwiches, 175
    Winemaker's Feast, The, 263
Portion control, gaining
    awareness of, 41
Portobello Stroganoff over
    Egg Noodles, 238
Potatoes
    Breakfast Burrito, 124–125
    Louisiana Shrimp Boil,
        249–251
    Niçoise-Style Salad, 132–134
    Vegetable Beef Stew, 230–231
Pot Roast with Sweet Potatoes, Peas,
    and Onions, 269–271
Poultry. See Chicken; Turkey
    in DASH diet, 45–46
Prediabetes, DASH diet and, 14–15
Progress, thinking, 50–51
Pumpkin seeds, Spice-Roasted
    Sunflower and, 187
Pureeing, 61

Q
Quesadillas, Tiny Turkey, 218–219
Quiche, Crustless Spinach, 114–115
Quick Vegetarian Ramen Noodle
    Soup, 226–227
Quinoa
    Pan-Seared Whitefish on
        Lemony Quinoa, 245
    Quinoa with Vegetables and
        Toasted Pecans, 156–157

R
Radishes
    Niçoise-Style Salad, 132–134
Raisins
    Sweet Potato Oatmeal, 100–101
Ramen noodles
    Quick Vegetarian Ramen
        Noodle Soup, 226–227

Raspberries
    Balsamic Berries, 288
    Berries in Meringue, 310
    Berry Apple Cobbler, 307
    Fruit Sauce for Sundaes, 284
    Vanilla and Lemon Berry
        Parfaits, 286–287
    Red, White, and Blue Fruit
        Kebabs, 186
    Rhubarb Compote, 285
Rice. See Brown rice; Saffron rice;
    Wild rice
Rice cakes
    Strawberry and Cream Cheese
        Cakes, 121
Ricotta cheese
    Cherries, Almonds, and
        Cheese, 281
    Cucumber and Ricotta Open-
        Face Sandwiches, 122
    Easy Breakfast Casserole with
        Vegetables, 113
    Frozen Chocolate Cannoli
        Sandwiches, 292
    Vegetable Lasagna, 239–241
Roasted Red Pepper Dip, 206–207
Roasted Vegetables on Ciabatta,
    154–155
Romaine lettuce
    Almost Mexican Pita, 150–151
    Cold Avocado and Shrimp
        Soup, 145
Roma tomatoes
    Coconut Fish Stew, 228
    Homemade Tomato Soup,
        142–143
    Tiny Turkey Quesadillas,
        218–219
    Vegetable Lasagna, 239–241
Rosemary
    Chicken Breasts with Mango-
        Rosemary Sauce on Brown
        Rice, 262
    Grilled Pork Tenderloin with
        Garlic and Herbs, 264–265
    Simple Rosemary Salmon,
        164–165
    Winemaker's Feast, The, 263

S
Saffron Rice, Lemon-Scented
    Chicken Kebabs on, 253–254
Salads
    Crunchy Chicken Salad, 140
    Flattened Chicken on Arugula
        Salad, 139
    Massaged Kale Salad, 138
    Niçoise-Style Salad, 132–134

Noodle Salad with Shrimp and
    Cucumber, 166
Orange, Avocado, and Shrimp
    Salad, 135
Substantial Fruit Salad, 98
Watermelon and Pistachio
    Salad, 202
Watermelon, Feta, and Mint
    Summer Salad, 136–167
Salmon
    Simple Rosemary Salmon,
        164–165
    Wild Salmon Salad Pita, 153
Salt, 16
    using spices instead of, 60
Sandwiches
    Cilantro-Avocado Tea
        Sandwiches, 213
    Cucumber and Dill Tea
        Sandwiches, 215
    Cucumber and Ricotta Open-
        Face Sandwiches, 122
    Frozen Chocolate Cannoli
        Sandwiches, 292
    Simple Lobster Tea
        Sandwiches, 214
    Vietnamese Pork
        Sandwiches, 175
    Watercress Tea Sandwiches
        with Sweet-Hot
        Mayonnaise, 212
Sardines, Hummus and,
    on Toast, 123
Scottish Meatloaf, 267
Searing
    Perfect Pan-Seared Fish,
        246–247
Seeds. See also Pumpkin seeds;
    Sunflower seeds
    in DASH diet, 45
    Granola, Your Way, 102
Shopping tips, for DASH diet,
    315–316
Shrimp
    Coconut Fish Stew, 228
    Cold Avocado and Shrimp
        Soup, 145
    Louisiana Shrimp Boil,
        249–251
    Noodle Salad with Shrimp and
        Cucumber, 166
    Orange, Avocado, and Shrimp
        Salad, 135
    Shrimp and Mango
        "Ceviche," 216
    Shrimp with Jalapeño-Orange
        Sauce over Pasta, 248
Simple Lobster Tea Sandwiches, 214
Simple Rosemary Salmon, 164–165

Smoothies
Green Monster, The, 92–93
Green Tea and Banana
Smoothie, 90
Mango Blast Smoothie, 88–89
Stomach Soother
Smoothie, The, 91
Vegetable Smoothie, 192–193
Snacks and appetizers, 183–223
Agua Fresca, 184–185
Baked Applesauce with
Walnuts, 199
Baked Chili-Lime Tortilla
Chips, 198
Cajun Popcorn, 191
Cilantro-Avocado Tea
Sandwiches, 213
Cucumber and Dill Tea
Sandwiches, 216
Cucumber Gazpacho, 194
DASH Meatballs, 222–223
Herbed Deviled Eggs, 210–211
Homemade Hummus with
Crudités, 209
Lemon-Glazed Tiny
Drumsticks, 220
Onion and Herb Dip, 204–205
Pickled Cucumbers, 195
Red, White, and Blue Fruit
Kebabs, 186
Roasted Red Pepper Dip,
206–207
Shrimp and Mango
"Ceviche," 216
Simple Lobster Tea
Sandwiches, 214
Spiced Edamame, 188–189
Spice-Roasted Sunflower and
Pumpkin Seeds, 187
Spicy Oil-Roasted
Chickpeas, 208
Strawberry-Mango Salsa with
Basil, 200–201
Sweet-Hot Maple Almond, 190
Thai Pork in Lettuce Wraps, 221
Tiny Turkey Quesadillas,
218–219
Tomato Salsa with Jalapeños
and Lime, 203
Turkey Mozzarella Shooters, 217
Vegetable Chips, 196–197
Vegetable Smoothie, 192–193
Watercress Tea Sandwiches
with Sweet-Hot
Mayonnaise, 212
Watermelon and Pistachio
Salad, 202

Soba noodles
Cold Soba Noodles with Peanut
Sauce, 160–161
Sodium, 6
reducing, in alleviating high
blood pressure, 19
smart choices for, 23
Soft Beef Tacos, 176–177
Soups
Coconut Soup, 289
Cold Avocado and Shrimp
Soup, 145
Cucumber Gazpacho, 194
Homemade Tomato Soup,
142–143
Melon Soup with Mint and
Yogurt, 144
Quick Vegetarian Ramen
Noodle Soup, 226–227
White Bean and Sage Soup, 141
Sour cream. See also Yogurt
Onion and Herb Dip, 204–205
Portobello Stroganoff over Egg
Noodles, 238
Roasted Red Pepper Dip,
206–207
Soy milk
Egg Tart with Sweet Potato
Crust, 118–120
Oatmeal with Pistachios and
Currants, 99
Soy Milk Shakes, 280
Spanish-Style Scrambled Eggs, 108
Special occasions, planning ahead
for, 50
Spiced Edamame, 188–189
Spice-Roasted Sunflower and
Pumpkin Seeds, 187
Spices, using instead of salt, 60
Spicy Chickpeas and Turkey,
167–168
Spicy Oil-Roasted Chickpeas, 208
Spicy Tofu Stir-Fry, 244
Spinach
Breakfast Burrito, 124–125
Creamy Beans and Greens, 232
Crustless Spinach Quiche,
114–115
Vegetable Smoothie, 192–193
Watermelon, Feta, and Mint
Summer Salad, 136–167
Spring greens
Mini Crab Cakes on Baby
Greens, 162–163
Squash
Layered Vegetable Casserole,
234

Vegetable Chips, 196–197
Vegetable Lasagna, 239–241
Steaming, 60
Stews
Coconut Fish Stew, 228
Vegetable Beef Stew, 230–231
Stir-fry
Lightning-Fast Chicken Stir-
Fry, 171
Spicy Tofu Stir-Fry, 244
Stomach Soother Smoothie, The, 91
Strawberries
Balsamic Berries, 288
Berries in Meringue, 310
Dark Chocolate–Covered
Fruits, 302
Fruit-Filled French Toast, 126
Fruit Sauce for Sundaes, 284
Peach Berry Fizz, 94
Red, White, and Blue Fruit
Kebabs, 186
Strawberry and Cream Cheese
Cakes, 121
Strawberry-Mango Salsa with
Basil, 200–201
Sweet Potato Oatmeal, 100–101
Vanilla and Lemon Berry
Parfaits, 286–287
Substantial Fruit Salad, 98
Success, steps for, 48–51
Sun-dried tomatoes
Onion and Herb Dip, 204–205
Sunflower seeds
Spice-Roasted Sunflower and
Pumpkin Seeds, 187
Sweet-Hot Maple Almond, 190
Sweet potatoes
Breakfast Hash, 127
Egg Tart with Sweet Potato
Crust, 118–120
Pot Roast with Sweet Potatoes,
Peas, and Onions, 269–271
Sweet Potato Oatmeal, 100–101
Vegetable Chips, 196–197
Sweet Potato Oatmeal, 100–101
Swiss cheese
Folded French Omelet,
104–105
Tiny Turkey Quesadillas,
218–219

T

Tacos, Soft Beef, 176–177
Tarragon
Hollywood Broiled
Grapefruit, 95

Tea and Jam Platter, 282–283
Temptation, eliminating
    undesirable, 39–41
Thai Pork in Lettuce Wraps, 221
30-day meal plan for health and
    weight loss, 62–84
Tiny Turkey Quesadillas, 218–219
Tofu, Spicy, Stir-Fry, 244
Tomatoes. *See also* Cherry
    tomatoes; Grape tomatoes;
    Roma tomatoes; Sun-dried
    tomatoes
    Almost Mexican Pita, 150–151
    Breakfast Burrito, 124–125
    Chicken Curry, 172–174
    Egg Tart with Sweet Potato
      Crust, 118–120
    Pasta Caprese, 158–159
    Quick Vegetarian Ramen
      Noodle Soup, 226–227
    Roasted Vegetables on Ciabatta,
      154–155
    Spicy Chickpeas and Turkey,
      167–168
    Tomato Salsa with Jalapeños
      and Lime, 203
    Turkey Bolognese, 242–243
    Turkey Chili with Black
      Beans, 229
    Vegetable and Hummus
      Pita, 152
    Vegetable Napoleons, 149
Tortillas
    Baked Chili-Lime Tortilla
      Chips, 198
    Breakfast Burrito, 124–125
    DASH Migas, 116
    Soft Beef Tacos, 176–177
    Tiny Turkey Quesadillas,
      218–219
Turkey
    Homemade Breakfast Sausage,
      Three Ways, 128–129
    Spicy Chickpeas and Turkey,
      167–168
    Tiny Turkey Quesadillas,
      218–219
    Turkey and Rice–Stuffed
      Peppers, 252
    Turkey Bolognese, 242–243
    Turkey Burgers with
      Cranberry-Scallion Sauce,
      169–170
    Turkey Chili with Black
      Beans, 229
    Turkey Mozzarella Shooters, 217
Turnips
    Vegetable Chips, 196–197

V

Vanilla and Lemon Berry Parfaits,
    286–287
Vegetable and Hummus Pita, 152
Vegetable and Mozzarella Frittata,
    146–148
Vegetable Beef Stew, 230–231
Vegetable Chips, 196–197
Vegetable Lasagna, 239–241
Vegetable Napoleons, 149
Vegetable proteins in DASH diet,
    45–46
Vegetables in DASH diet, 44
Vegetable Smoothie, 192–193
Vietnamese Pork Sandwiches, 175

W

Walnuts
    Baked Applesauce with
      Walnuts, 199
    Heart-Healing Chocolate Chip
      Cookies, 298–300
Watercress
    Onion and Herb Dip, 204–205
    Watercress Tea Sandwiches
      with Sweet-Hot
      Mayonnaise, 212
Watermelon
    Agua Fresca, 164–165
    Watermelon and Pistachio
      Salad, 202
    Watermelon, Feta, and Mint
      Summer Salad, 136–167
    Watermelon Ice, 274–275
Weight, determining your, 36–37
Weight loss
    DASH diet for, 24–29
    30-day meal plan for, 62–84
Wheat germ
    Oatmeal with Pistachios and
      Currants, 99
    Sweet Potato Oatmeal, 100–101
White Bean and Sage Soup, 141
Whole-wheat bread
    Cilantro-Avocado Tea
      Sandwiches, 213
    Cucumber and Dill Tea
      Sandwiches, 215
    Simple Lobster Tea
      Sandwiches, 214
    Vietnamese Pork
      Sandwiches, 175
    Watercress Tea Sandwiches
      with Sweet-Hot
      Mayonnaise, 212

Whole-wheat flour
    Berry Apple Cobbler, 307
    Chocolate Olive Oil Cake, 314
    Clafouti, 306
    Lighten Up Brownies, 308–309
Wild Rice, Chicken Breast with
    Mushroom Sauce on, 260–261
Wild Salmon Salad Pita, 153
Winemaker's Feast, The, 263
Wrapping, 61
Wraps, Thai Pork in Lettuce, 221

Y

Yogurt. *See also* Sour cream
    Acorn Squash, Apple, and Peach
      "Pie," 103
    Balsamic Berries, 288
    Coconut Soup, 289
    Cucumber Gazpacho, 194
    Fruit-Filled French Toast, 126
    Grilled Peaches, 304–305
    Hollywood Broiled
      Grapefruit, 95
    Homemade Tomato Soup,
      142–143
    Mango Blast Smoothie, 88–89
    Melon Soup with Mint and
      Yogurt, 144
    Onion and Herb Dip, 204–205
    Pears Poached in Orange Juice
      and Red Wine, 303
    Soy Milk Shakes, 280
    Stomach Soother
      Smoothie, The, 91
    Substantial Fruit Salad, 98
    Vanilla and Lemon Berry
      Parfaits, 286–287
    Vegetable Smoothie, 192–193
    Yogurt and Tropical Fruit
      Parfaits, 96–97

Z

Zucchini
    Layered Vegetable
      Casserole, 234
    Quick Vegetarian Ramen
      Noodle Soup, 226–227
    Quinoa with Vegetables and
      Toasted Pecans, 156–157
    Vegetable Chips, 196–197
    Vegetable Lasagna, 239–241
    Vegetable Napoleons, 149

CPSIA information can be obtained at www.ICGtesting.com
Printed in the USA
BVOW10s2219171013

334029BV00001B/1/P